Essentials in Ophthalmology

Series Editor
Arun D. Singh

For further volumes:
http://www.springer.com/series/5332

Hakan Demirci

Editor

Arun D. Singh
Series Editor

Orbital Inflammatory Diseases and Their Differential Diagnosis

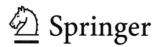

Editor
Hakan Demirci, MD
Ophthalmology and Visual Sciences
W.K. Kellogg Eye Center
Ann Arbor, MI
USA

Series Editor
Arun D. Singh
Department of Ophthalmic Oncology
Cole Eye Institute
Cleveland Clinic Foundation
Cleveland, OH
USA

ISSN 1612-3212   ISSN 2196-890X   (electronic)
Essentials in Ophthalmology
ISBN 978-3-662-46527-1   ISBN 978-3-662-46528-8   (eBook)
DOI 10.1007/978-3-662-46528-8

Library of Congress Control Number: 2015936587

Springer Heidelberg New York Dordrecht London
© Springer-Verlag Berlin Heidelberg 2015

Printed on acid-free paper

Springer-Verlag GmbH Berlin Heidelberg is part of Springer Science+Business Media
(www.springer.com)

Preface

Recent advances in genetics and molecular biology have significantly increased the understanding of inflammatory disorders, which allows for more accurate diagnosis and provide better care for orbital inflammatory disorders. Orbital inflammatory disorders are common, but relatively less-known. There are few books that provide in-depth and up-to-date information about orbital inflammatory disorders. This book summarizes the recent developments on the spectrum of orbital inflammatory disorders in a concise and thorough manner. Newly introduced IgG4-related orbital inflammation, developments in pathogenesis, management of thyroid eye disease, and orbital xanthogranulomatous disorders are recent advancements that are reviewed in this book. This reference book will be useful for ophthalmology residents, general ophthalmologists, oculoplastics and orbital surgeons, ocular oncologists, otolaryngologists, and neurosurgeons during their daily practice for patient care. Additionally, its easy-to-read style makes this book a valuable source for examination review and updating knowledge of orbital inflammatory disorders.

I would like to sincerely thank all of the contributing authors, Victor M. Elner, Raymond S. Douglas, Adam S. Hassan, Gangadhara Sundar, Santosh Honavar, Shivani Gupta, Zachary D. Pearce, Sima Das, and Shannon S. Joseph, for their thorough review of topics. Also, I thank Dr. Arun Singh and Tracy Marton for their help with editing. Finally, I would like to thank my family for their continuous support in my endeavors over the years.

Ann Arbor, MI, USA   Hakan Demirci, MD

Contents

Orbital Infections

Sima Das and Santosh G. Honavar

1.1 Introduction

Infections of the orbit are caused by a wide variety of microorganisms. The anatomic position of the orbit in the face makes it susceptible to involvement by contiguous spread of the infection from the surrounding structures [1]. Orbital infections usually present as an acute orbital inflammation; however, a chronic indolent presentation, mimicking neoplastic orbital processes, can be seen in cases of the fungal infections. Bacterial aetiology is the most common case of orbital infection. Fungal and parasitic infections can also involve the orbit. This chapter discusses the clinical manifestations, microbiological profile, management outline and complications of bacterial, fungal and parasitic infections of the orbit.

S. Das, MD
Oculoplasty and Ocular Oncology Services
Department, Dr Shroff's Charity Eye Hospital,
New Delhi 110002, India
e-mail: contactsima@gmail.com

S.G. Honavar, MD (✉)
Ophthalmic and Facial Plastic Surgery
and Ocular Oncology Department, Centre for Sight
Eye Hospital, Road No 2, Banjara Hills, Hyderabad,
Telangana 500034, India
e-mail: santosh.honavar@gmail.com

1.2 Bacterial Orbital Infections

Bacterial infection of the orbit is primarily a disease of the children and young adults with peak incidence reported in 0–15 years age group [2, 3]. It usually presents as an acute orbit and is considered one of the medical emergencies. Paranasal sinus disease is the most common predisposing factor both in children and adults. Ethmoid sinus infection most commonly involves the orbit by contiguous spread as the thin bony medial wall of the orbit and the presence of numerous foramina and valveless venous connections allow for ready spread of the infection to the orbit [4–6]. Contiguous infections of the eyelids and orbit like stye, dacryocystitis, dacryoadenitis, canaliculitis, panophthalmitis and infections of the face like furuncle can spread to the orbit and cause orbital cellulitis. Other sources of orbital infection are post trauma, orbital foreign body, dental abscess, postorbital surgery and upper respiratory tract infection [2, 5, 7, 8].

Microbiological profile of bacterial orbital infection depends on the age of the patient and the aetiology of the infection [2, 5]. In children, the most common organisms isolated are *Staphylococcus aureus*, *Streptococcus pneumoniae* and other streptococcus species [5, 9, 10]. *Haemophilus influenzae* was the most common organism in the era before the universal *Haemophilus influenzae type b* vaccination [9–11]. Widespread use of the vaccine has led to a considerable decline in the infection

H. Demirci (ed.), *Orbital Inflammatory Diseases and Their Differential Diagnosis*,
Essentials in Ophthalmology, DOI 10.1007/978-3-662-46528-8_1,
© Springer-Verlag Berlin Heidelberg 2015

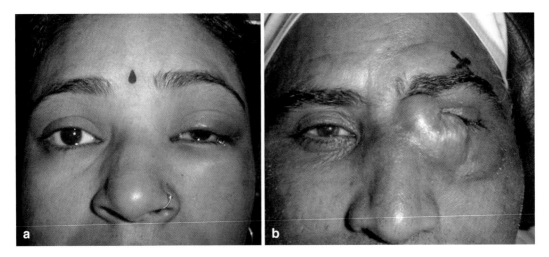

Fig. 1.1 Preseptal cellulitis in young adult secondary to hordeolum externum (**a**) and acute dacryocystitis (**b**)

caused by this organism [12, 13]. The incidence of orbital infection caused by methicillin-resistant *Staphylococcus aureus* (MRSA) has seen an increased trend recently, and hence empirical antibiotic therapy should be directed towards these organisms especially if it is prevalent in the community [5, 14]. Polymicrobial infections are seen more commonly in adults [2]. Organisms can be isolated from culture of the exudates obtained by surgical intervention from affected sinus or abscess cavity or from conjunctival swab culture. Blood cultures are rarely positive. Orbital infection caused by *Pseudomonas aeruginosa* and *Proteus mirabilis* has been reported in association with systemic bacteraemia in patients with diabetes mellitus, acute leukaemia and cholecystitis and in association with endophthalmitis following cataract surgery [15, 16]. Other rare organisms reported to cause orbital infection are *Bacillus thuringiensis*, *Arcanobacterium haemolyticum* and *Kingella kingae* in paediatric patients and *Yersinia enterocolitica* in case of post-traumatic orbital cellulitis [17–20].

Paranasal sinus disease remains the most common predisposing cause for orbital infection, and the orbital complications of sinusitis have been described by Smith and Spencer and modified by Chandler [21, 22]. This classification system defines the severity and location of the disease process, although disease progression does not always occur according to the described stages.

1.2.1 Preseptal Cellulitis

In preseptal cellulitis, the infection is limited to the skin and subcutaneous tissues anterior to the orbital septum. Clinically, it presents as a rapidly progressive eyelid oedema and erythema with or without conjunctival congestion and chemosis, commonly in children (Fig. 1.1). There is absence of proptosis and pupillary dysfunction, and ocular movements are unaffected which differentiates this disease process from orbital cellulitis. Skin infection and upper respiratory tract infection are common predisposing factors for the development of preseptal cellulitis in children. Trauma, hordeolum externum, acute dacryocystitis, conjunctivitis and sinusitis are other predisposing factors both in children and adults.

The common organisms causing preseptal cellulitis in children include *Streptococcus pneumoniae*, *Staphylococcus* species and *Haemophilus influenzae* [3, 5]. The causative organism can be isolated by culturing the abscess material. Blood culture is indicated in acutely ill children with high fever, and suspected septicaemia though a positive yield is rare. Recently, MRSA has emerged as the most common causative organism in preseptal and orbital cellulitis [2, 14, 23]. Preseptal cellulitis needs to be differentiated from other causes of periocular swelling like allergic periocular oedema, angioneurotic oedema, thyroid eye disease, etc.

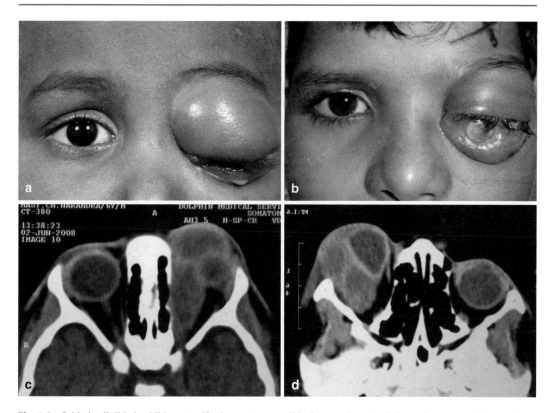

Fig. 1.2 Orbital cellulitis in children manifesting as tense eyelid edema and proptosis (**a**) and severe proptosis and corneal exposure (**b**). CT scan showing large subperiosteal (**c**) and intraorbital abscess (**d**) requiring immediate drainage

Bacteremic preseptal cellulitis is commonly treated with parenteral antibiotics. The initial choice of antibiotic can be decided by the Gram stain and microscopy results and modified based on the culture sensitivity reports. Non-vaccine strains of *Streptococcus pneumoniae* are the common cause of the infection in children; hence, empirical antibiotic therapy should include a third-generation cephalosporin. Hospitalisation and inpatient treatment and monitoring for the development of a life-threatening complication like meningitis are preferred in infants and neonates as their immune systems are less effective against encapsulated bacterial infection [24]. Older children and adults can be treated with oral antibiotics on an outpatient basis. Orbital spread of preseptal infection is associated with worsening of symptoms, onset of proptosis and restriction of ocular movements. Orbital imaging is indicated in patients with suspected orbital cellulitis or patients with worsening of symptoms despite continued systemic antibiotic treatment. Computed tomography (CT) scan of orbits is done to rule out orbital abscess or any occult foreign body in the setting of trauma. Non-response to treatment also calls for revaluation of the antibiotic sensitivity in patients with positive culture material. Surgical management is indicated for abscess drainage and removal of foreign body in post-trauma cases. Abscess cavity is irrigated with antibiotic solution and the wound left open for exudates to drain.

1.2.2   Orbital Cellulitis

The clinical features of orbital cellulitis include pain, eyelid oedema and erythema, conjunctival congestion and chemosis and signs of involvement of postseptal orbit like presence of proptosis and ocular motility restriction which differentiated this from preseptal cellulitis (Fig. 1.2). Afferent pupillary defect and other signs of optic nerve compression may be present in cases with orbital or subperiosteal abscess. Sinusitis is the most common predisposing factor for the development of orbital cellulitis both in children and adults [2, 5]. Other predisposing causes are trauma with orbital foreign body inoculation, dental abscess, dacryocystitis and systemic conditions like diabetes mellitus [25, 26]. Sinus infection, especially ethmoid sinusitis, can spread to the orbit readily due to the thin wall of the lamina papyracea and presence of several foramina and natural dehiscences which provide a ready communication between the orbit and sinus.

In patients with positive culture, *Staphylococcus aureus* has been identified as the most common aetiologic agent in adult patients with orbital cellulitis. In children, various species of *Streptococcus* have been reported as the most common pathogen. Other reported causative organisms include *Haemophilus influenzae*, *Corynebacterium*, *Clostridium*, *Enterococcus*, *Pseudomonas* and anaerobes.

The clinical features of the orbital cellulitis associated with sinusitis have been described by Smith and Spencer and modified later by Chandler [21, 22]. This classification is based on the severity of the disease process. Class I is inflammatory preseptal eyelid swelling associated with sinusitis, possibly due to congestion of the orbital venous drainage system. There are no other signs of orbital involvement like proptosis and ophthalmoplegia at this stage. In class II, there is involvement of the orbit as suggested clinically by the presence of proptosis, ophthalmoplegia and signs of optic nerve compression. Radiologically, orbital involvement can be seen as streaking of the orbital fat and diffuse soft tissue thickening on CT scan. Localised collection of the purulent material from the sinus can occur in the subperiosteal space (class III) or into the orbit (class IV). Orbital abscess is diagnosed on imaging and appears as a hypodense collection along the orbital walls or into the extra- and intraconal spaces. Presence of orbital abscess is suspected in patients with non-respose to treatment or worsening of signs and symptoms with increase in pain, tenderness and tense orbit with motility restriction and possible decreased vision

with signs of optic nerve compression. Cavernous sinus involvement can occur due to the posterior spread of the infection through the venous system and is the most serious complication of orbital cellulitis (class V). Onset of cavernous sinus thrombosis is associated with high fever with or without signs of CNS involvement like altered sensorium, onset of contralateral eyelid oedema and skin discoloration, contralateral ophthalmoplegia and extraocular muscle paresis and proptosis. MRI is indicated to confirm the diagnosis of cavernous sinus thrombosis. Absence of flow or luminal narrowing on T2-weighted and gadolinium-enhanced images will confirm the diagnosis.

Orbital cellulitis is an ophthalmic emergency, and management needs hospitalisation and treatment with intravenous antibiotics with close monitoring to identify and treat any complication at the earliest. Initial empirical antibiotic chosen should cover a broad spectrum of bacteria including *Staphylococcus*, *Streptococcus* and anaerobes. Third-generation cephalosporins or ampicillin-sulbactam combinations are initial antibiotics of choice. If anaerobic infection is suspected, metronidazole or clindamycin can be added. The antibiotic can be changed based on the sensitivity report if a specific positive culture is available and a specific organism is isolated. The optimal duration of antibiotic treatment is variable with 14–21 days being the minimal suggested duration as with other severe infections like meningitis [5]. Imaging modality like CT scan is indicated to rule out orbital abscess, sinusitis or orbital foreign body in the setting of trauma. The patient is sent for the imaging after giving the initial dose of antibiotic. Subperiosteal orbital abscess associated with sinusitis needs surgical drainage if signs of compressive optic neuropathy are present or no improvement in signs and symptoms is noted after 24–48 hours of antibiotic therapy. Young patients with small medial subperiosteal abscess without any signs of complication can be managed medically, while large abscess needs drainage [27]. Abscess along the medial orbital wall can be drained either by endonasal or orbital route. Endonasal route is preferred if associated ethmoid sinus collection also needs drainage [28].

Orbital route is preferred for drainage along the other orbital walls. Though the decision to drain subperiosteal abscess is ultimately guided by the clinical course, the volume of the abscess material as determined on CT scan has been found to correlate with the need for drainage with subperiosteal abscess more than 1,250 mm requiring drainage in a study by Todman and Enzer [29]. Orbital abscess with collection of pus within intra- or extraconal space needs immediate drainage as the inflammatory and infectious collections release mediators which are toxic to orbital tissues. Orbital cellulitis associated with retained wooden or vegetative foreign body in post-trauma cases requires orbital surgery for foreign body removal.

1.3 Fungal Orbital Infection

Fungal infections of the orbit are relatively rare and can mimic other infectious, inflammatory and neoplastic conditions of the orbit, thereby delaying the diagnosis in some cases. Though a variety of fungus can invade the orbit, the main aetiologic organisms causing invasive orbital infection include *Rhizopus*, *Mucor*, *Absidia* and *Aspergillus* species [30]. Because of the proximity of the orbit to the paranasal sinuses, fungal orbital infections are usually acquired by extension of paranasal sinus disease [31]. Direct implantation of the organism to the orbit can occur following trauma. Infection can also spread to the orbit from a distant site by haematogenous route.

1.3.1 Mucormycosis

Mucormycosis or zygomycosis is an acute fulminant fungal infection caused by the *Rhizopus*, *Mucor* and *Absidia* species. It is usually found in immunocompromised patients with diabetic ketoacidosis being the most important risk factor [32]. Other risk factors include immunosuppression in cases of bone marrow transplantation intravenous drug use, long-term corticosteroid therapy, desferrioxamine therapy and neutropenia [30, 33]. Mucormycosis is rarely reported in immunocompetent patients. The infection is usually acquired by colonisation of the nasal and oral mucosa by the fungal spores which spread to the paranasal sinus and orbit.

The clinical presentation is usually acute with fever, periorbital pain and inflammation, epistaxis, ptosis, ophthalmoplegia, proptosis, loss of corneal sensation and decreased vision (Fig. 1.3). The extent of cranial nerve paresis is usually out of proportion to the amount of inflammation which provides a clue to the diagnosis. The organism has the propensity for angioinvasion which can cause vascular occlusion and ischemic tissue necrosis which adds to the area of the septic necrosis caused by the fungus. Tissue infarction and necrosis also cause the typical black-coloured eschar over the palate, nasal septum and facial skin which are usually the late manifestations of the infection. Invasion and occlusion of the central retinal artery or choroidal vasculature is responsible for the early and severe visual loss.

Extension of the disease can occur from the sinus to the orbit and to the brain through orbital apex, cribriform plate or via blood vessels [34]. Rhino-orbital-cerebral mucormycosis can be a fatal disease if not treated, and early diagnosis and prompt management are imperative to reduce the mortality and morbidity associated with the disease. Imaging the orbit and paranasal sinuses with CT or MRI is indicated in uncontrolled diabetic or immunocompromised patients with acute onset of ophthalmoplegia, proptosis and decreased vision to rule out mucormycosis. CT scan reveals opacification of the sinus by the mass, bone erosion and extension to the orbit. Early CT findings are thickening of the extraocular muscles adjacent to the involved sinus [35]. Diagnosis is confirmed by KOH mount, *Gomori's* methenamine silver stain and culture of the biopsy material obtained from the eschar material or paranasal sinus or orbital mass. The fungus is seen as large, right angle branching, nonseptate hyphae on smear.

The management approach for orbital mucormycosis includes an early diagnosis and prompt institution of systemic antifungal therapy. Polyene antifungal amphotericin B administered intravenously is the drug of choice. The drug is

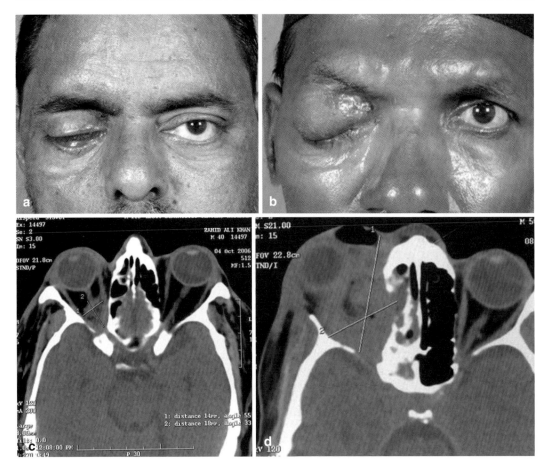

Fig. 1.3 Orbital mucormycosis presenting as total ophthalmoplegia with orbital inflammation (**a**) and with associated eyelid skin fistulae (**b**) in patients with uncontrolled diabetes. CT scan showing opacification near the orbital apex and associated extraocular muscle thickening (**c**) and diffuse orbital and ethmoid sinus involvement (**d**)

potentially nephrotoxic and hence needs dose titration and monitoring of the renal functions. Liposomal amphotericin B has less nephrotoxicity with good tissue penetration and is an alternative to amphotericin B [30, 35]. However, the preparation is more expensive compared to amphotericin B. A newer antifungal like posaconazole is better tolerated than amphotericin B and can be an alternative in patients not tolerating or responding to amphotericin B [36]. Extensive surgical debridement is needed in most patients to remove the necrosed tissue and allow for the penetration of antifungal medications. Surgical procedure can range from drainage and aeration of the involved sinuses to radical orbital exenteration. Local irrigation with amphotericin B following surgical debridement is also advocated in

few studies [37]. Urgent neurosurgical consultation is needed in patients with CNS involvement. Hyperbaric oxygen therapy is also shown to be effective in the treatment of mucormycosis as it decreases the local acidosis which promotes fungal growth [38].Control of the underlying condition like diabetic ketoacidosis or systemic immunosuppression is of utmost importance for controlling the infection.

1.3.2 Orbital Aspergillosis

Aspergillus infection of the orbit can occur in two different clinical forms, invasive and non-invasive orbital infection [39]. Invasive orbital aspergillosis usually occurs in immu-

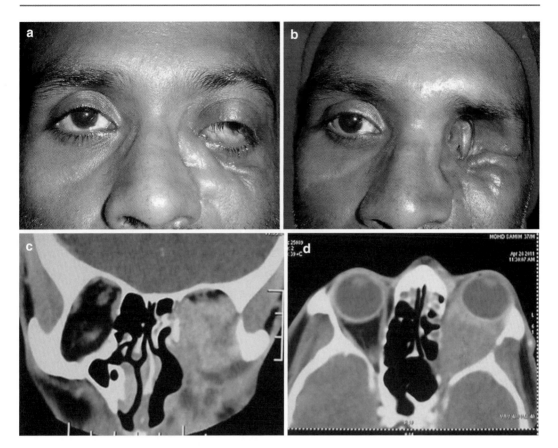

Fig. 1.4 Pre- (**a**) and postoperative (**b**) photographs of a young adult with recurrent invasive sino-orbital aspergillosis status post debridement managed by orbital exenteration, partial maxillectomy and systemic voriconazole. CT scan shows extensive sino-orbital mass filling the maxillary sinus and orbit and extending to the orbital apex (**c**, **d**)

nocompromised patients, and the predisposing factors are similar to that of mucormycosis infection. The presentation can be acute with clinical picture resembling orbital cellulitis with proptosis, ptosis, ophthalmoplegia and visual loss (Fig. 1.4). Vascular invasion can cause tissue ischemia, and the black eschar characteristic of mucormycosis can also be seen in the late stages of *Aspergillus* infection [39]. *Aspergillus* have propensity to involve the sphenoid sinus more commonly probably due to the hypoxic environment, and this can present as optic neuropathy without other signs of orbital involvement [30]. A non-invasive form of orbital aspergillosis occurs usually in immunocompetent patients as an extension from the sinus disease, commonly maxillary sinus disease. The disease is commonly caused by *Aspergillus fumigatus* and starts with colonisation and expansion of the sinus cavity. Breakdown of the anatomical barrier causes orbital extension of the disease. The symptoms are primarily due to pressure effect by orbital mass and present as slowly progressive proptosis with globe displacement.

CT scan is the diagnostic investigation of choice if sino-orbital aspergillosis is suspected. The infection appears as heterogeneous opacification of the sinus with the presence of calcification which is highly suggestive of *Aspergillus* infection. Focal areas of bone destruction can be seen on CT. In early stages of the disease, severe unilateral thickening of the nasal mucosa on CT scan is found to be a consistent finding and should raise suspicion of invasive fungal infection [40]. Diagnosis is confirmed by endoscopic biopsy and

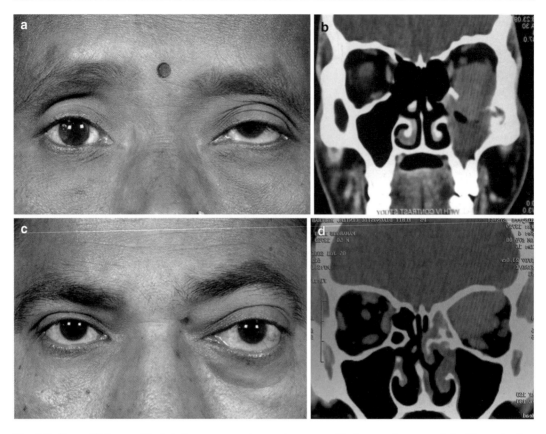

Fig. 1.5 Sino-orbital aspergillosis in immunocompetent patients. Proptosis with superior globe displacement (**a**) caused by maxillary sinus aspergillosis causing orbital floor destruction and extending to the orbit (**b**). Ethmoid sinus aspergillosis extending to medial orbit causing lateral globe displacement (**c**). In addition to the ethmoid sinus mass, note thickening of the ipsilateral nasal mucosa on CT scan (**d**)

microscopy and culture of the involved sinus tissue or orbital mass. Microscopy of the KOH-mounted tissue can provide a rapid diagnosis about the type of fungus but cannot provide information about tissue invasion. It is important to take superficial and deep biopsies and send the material for histopathology and special staining with *Gomori's* methenamine silver and periodic acid-Schiff to avoid false negative results and to detect invasive disease which will help in deciding about the management option [41].

Non-invasive sino-orbital aspergillosis is usually treated by surgical debridement of the orbital mass and the involved sinuses. Antifungal therapy is usually not indicated, and prognosis remains good in these cases. Invasive sino-orbital aspergillosis is a potentially fatal disease, and urgent treatment is indicated with a combination of surgical debridement and systemic antifungal therapy (Fig. 1.5). The involved sinus and orbital tissues are debrided and aerated. Orbital exenteration might be needed in cases with extensive orbital involvement; especially with involvement of the orbital apex to prevent intracerebral spread of the infection [41]. Intravenous amphotericin B is the mainstay medical treatment. Liposomal amphotericin B is better tolerated and more effective and with lower renal toxicity compared to amphotericin B. Irrigation of the sinus and orbital cavity can be done with amphotericin B during the time of debridement. Recently, a new azole group of drug, voriconazole, has been approved by FDA as the first-line treatment for invasive sino-orbital aspergillosis. This drug is well tolerated with minimal side effects like visual disturbance and skin rash [42]. In immunocompromised patients, particular attention should be paid to reverse the predisposing factor. Complication includes involvement of the cavernous sinus and cerebrum involvement which is the cause of mortality in these patients.

1.4 Parasitic Orbital Infections

Parasitic infection of the orbit is uncommon compared to the bacterial and fungal infections. The common parasites causing orbital infection are cysticercosis and echinococcosis. Orbital diclofilariasis and myasis have also been reported rarely.

1.4.1 Orbital Cysticercosis

Orbital cysticercosis is caused by the *Cysticercus cellulosae*, the larval form of *Taenia solium*. In cysticercosis, the human being acts as the intermediate host, and the disease is acquired in humans by ingestion of the eggs through contaminated food, water or through autoinfection. Neurocysticercosis is the most common form of infection, and ocular involvement has been reported in 12.8–40 % cases [43, 44]. Intraocular cysticercosis has been thought to be the most common form of ocular involvement. However, recent studies have reported an increased incidence of adnexal and orbital disease, probably attributed to the increased awareness about the various clinical manifestations and availability of various imaging modalities like ultrasound B scan and CT scan which can detect the parasitic involvement of the various ocular structures [45]. Orbital cysticercosis is a disease of young adults and children with the median age reported as 13 years [46]. Males and females are affected equally.

Ocular motility restriction and proptosis are the most common clinical manifestations of the disease. Diplopia due to ocular movement restriction, pain and redness is the common presenting complaint. Other presentations include ptosis and eyelid and subconjunctival nodules. The clinical presentation can mimic orbital inflammatory disease or oculomotor nerve paresis [47, 48]. The anterior orbit is involved more commonly than the posterior orbit, and the cyst is found in relation to the extraocular muscle in 80 % cases. The medial rectus muscle is involved most commonly [49]. The toxin released by the dying parasite can induce an inflammatory response and can manifest as eyelid oedema and orbital cellulitis. Rarely, the bony orbit or subperiosteal space can be the primary site of involvement [50, 51]. Optic nerve involvement can present as primary optic neuritis or disc oedema causing diminished vision. The lacrimal gland can be involved rarely manifesting as dacryoadenitis [52].

Diagnosis of orbital cysticercosis is made based on the clinical features and imaging findings. History of recurrent orbital inflammation with remissions or acquired ptosis and proptosis with extraocular motility restriction in a young adult, especially in endemic areas, should raise a suspicion of orbital cysticercosis (Figs. 1.6 and 1.7). Blood investigations can reveal eosinophilia and serological test like ELISA for cysticercosis have a reported sensitivity of 65–98 % and specificity of 70–100 % [53]. Hence results of serological tests should be interpreted in the context of the clinical picture. Orbital imaging with ultrasound or CT scan is the most definitive diagnostic modality. On B scan ultrasound, a live cyst appears as sonolucent cavity with well-defined margins. The scolex within the cyst appears as a highly reflective spot within the cyst [54]. The response to the therapy and various stages of degradation of the cyst can be detected on ultrasound as regression in the size of the cyst, loss of the scolex, collapse of the walls and decrease in the muscle thickness [45]. On CT scan, the cyst appears isodense with the vitreous. Inflammatory response in case of a dying cyst can appear as contrast enhancement of the tissues around the cyst. B scan ultrasound is comparable to CT scan in detecting the cyst [45]. B scan has been reported to have a better ability to detect the scolex within the cyst as compared to CT scan. B scan can be the imaging modality of choice for serial imaging during the course of treatment as it is less expansive and avoids radiation exposure to the patient. However, during initial diagnosis, CT scan might be indicated to rule out any concurrent neurocysticercosis.

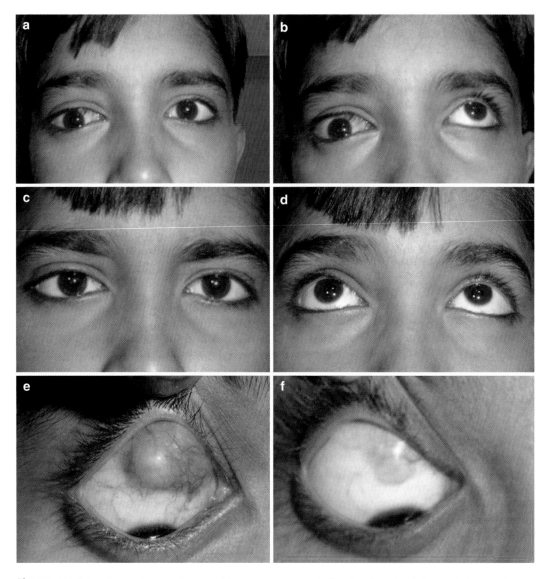

Fig. 1.6 Orbital cysticercosis presenting as sudden onset proptosis, strabismus and ocular motility restriction in a child (**a**, **b**). Resolution of proptosis and strabismus and improvement of ocular motility (**c**, **d**) following 4-week course of albendazole and oral steroid. Anterior extension of the cysticercus cyst is visible subconjunctivally (**e**) and responded well to medical management (**f**)

Medical therapy with oral antihelminthic and steroid remains the effective first line of management modality for orbital cysticercosis. Albendazole, administered at a dose of 15 mg/kg body weight, is the drug of choice [55]. Systemic prednisolone at a dose of 1 mg/kg body weight is administered concurrently to suppress the inflammation caused by the dying cyst. The treatment with oral antihelminthics is continued for 4–6 weeks. The response to therapy is judged by the resolution of symptoms like proptosis, ptosis and control of inflammation. The therapy can also be tailor-made based on the ultrasound findings, and antihelminthics can be discontinued once the scolex disappears on serial ultrasound [45]. Praziquantel is an alternative antihelminthic but is reported to be less effective than albendazole. Surgical excision of orbital cyst is rarely indi-

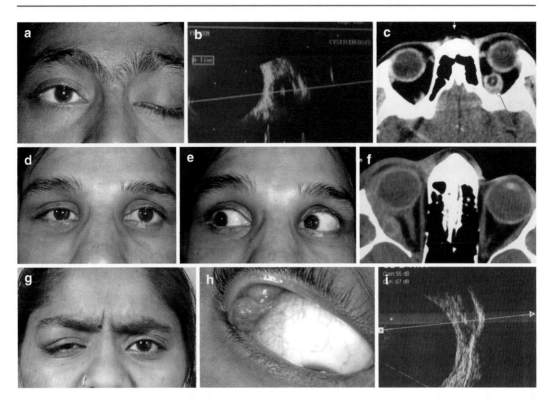

Fig. 1.7 Clinical presentation of orbital cysticercosis. Sudden onset ptosis in a 25-year-old male (**a**). Ultrasound B scan and CT scan showing well-defined cystic lesion in relation to superior rectus levator complex with hyperdense scolex within (**b**, **c**). Cysticercosis of lateral rectus presenting as painful acquired sixth nerve paresis (**d**, **e**). CT scan demonstrating lateral rectus thickening with hypodense area within suggestive of dying cyst with surrounding inflammation (**f**). Right acute dacryoadenitis in a young female patient (**g**) caused by lacrimal gland cysticercosis (**h**) detected by ultrasound B scan (**i**)

cated as the extensive dissection needed might induce further inflammation and fibrosis of the extraocular muscles and other orbital tissues. It is reserved for symptomatic patients with orbital or subconjunctival cysticercosis not responding to medical therapy.

1.4.2   Orbital Echinococcosis

Echinococcosis is a zoonotic disease and human involvement is caused by the larval stage of the genus *Echinococcus*. The four species which have been reported to cause human infestation are *Echinococcus granulosus* which causes cystic echinococcosis, *Echinococcus multilocularis* which causes alveolar echinococcosis and *Echinococcus oligarthrus* and *Echinococcus vogeli* which cause polycystic echinococcosis

[56, 57]. Dogs and wild animals are the definitive host, and the human acts as the intermediate host. The disease is endemic in those parts of the world where cattle and dogs are bred simultaneously and is acquired by ingestion of food contaminated with canine faeces containing the larvae of the organism. Orbital involvement is seen in 1–2 % cases, and in endemic areas orbital echinococcosis has been reported to be responsible for 5–20 % cases of all orbital mass lesion [58–61].

Painless progressive proptosis is the most common clinical presentation. Mass effect of the enlarging cyst on the orbital structures can cause optic nerve compression and globe displacement and luxation resulting in phthisis bulbi in late stages (Fig. 1.8). Rupture of the cyst can cause pain, increased proptosis and orbital inflammation [62, 63]. On CT scan, the lesion appears as hypodense well-defined single or multiple orbital

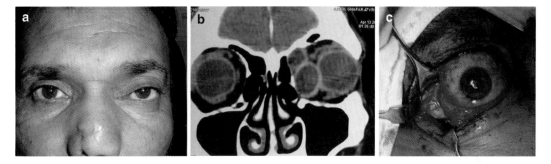

Fig. 1.8 Orbital hydatid cyst in a middle-aged male patient presenting as slowly progressive proptosis and globe displacement (**a**). CT scan shows well-defined, multilobed, cystic lesion in medial orbit suggestive of hydatid cyst (**b**). Intraoperative appearance of the white ectocyst capsule (**c**)

cyst. Orbital expansion due to pressure effect can be noted on CT scan. Localised condensation in the cyst wall can be noted in some cases which correspond to the area of collection of the scolices [63]. Haematological investigations can reveal eosinophilia and increased ESR. This coupled with the clinical findings, and CT appearance, especially in patients coming from endemic areas, will establish the diagnosis in most cases. Serological tests have high false negative values and are not very helpful for establishing the diagnosis [64].

Surgical cyst excision remains the treatment of choice though medical management with oral albendazole has been reported to cause reduction of the orbital cyst and resolution of non-ocular hydatid cyst [65, 66]. Preoperatively, albendazole is given in a dose of 15–30 mg/Kg body weight for 4–8 weeks, with 2-week interval in between. Oral antihelminthic treatment has also been recommended postoperatively following cyst excision. Transcutaneous injection of cysticidal agents like 30 % hypertonic saline and ethanol without any open surgery can be successful in some cases [67]. Surgical excision is associated with a high possibility of cyst rupture, and it is recommended to do an endocystectomy first and take out the cyst capsule later to prevent leakage of the cyst content into the orbit. The orbit is irrigated with hypertonic saline at the end of the procedure. Intraoperative cyst rupture can cause dissemination of the cyst and increased incidence of recurrence. The diagnosis is confirmed by histopathological evaluation of the excised cyst which shows a PAS-positive outer laminated membrane and inner membrane with brood capsules and protoscolices attached to it.

1.5 Orbital Tuberculosis

Orbital tuberculosis is a rare form of extrapulmonary tuberculosis and involves the orbit either by haematogenous dissemination of the systemic infection or by contiguous spread from the surrounding structures. The orbital soft tissues or bone or both can be involved primarily. The incidence of extrapulmonary tuberculosis has increased in the recent years with the advent of HIV infection. Based on the clinical presentation, the orbital tuberculosis can be divided into the following five categories: (1) periostitis, (2) orbital tuberculoma or cold abscess with no bone involvement, (3) orbital tuberculosis with bone involvement, (4) orbital spread from paranasal sinus tuberculosis and (5) dacryoadenitis [68].

Involvement of the orbital periosteum by tuberculosis usually presents as chronic discharging sinus or ulceration in the periorbital region (Fig. 1.9). The skin surrounding the sinus is often thickened, oedematous and adherent to the underlying bone and can have cicatricial ectropion. The orbital rim is most frequently involved, and CT scan shows variable degree of bone erosion, thickening and lysis.

Soft tissue involvement of the orbit can present as a tuberculoma or cold abscess and manifest as proptosis, orbital mass and extraocular motility disturbance. Compression effect on the globe and

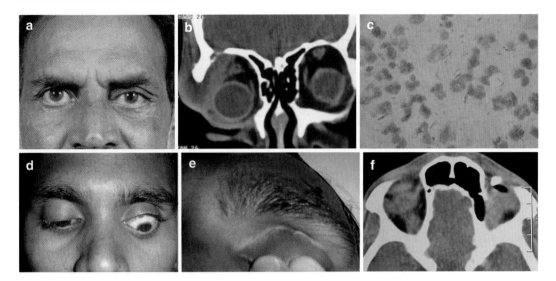

Fig. 1.9 Clinical manifestations of orbital tuberculosis. Progressive proptosis with lateral orbital mass in an elderly patient with history of fever and recent weight loss (**a**). Imaging showed a mixed density mass in lacrimal gland region with associated bone destruction (**b**). FNAB from orbital mass revealed numerous acid-fast bacilli suggestive of orbital tuberculosis (**c**). Tuberculosis of the orbital bone presenting as cicatricial lagophthalmos and eyelid retraction with fistulae formation in a young male (**d**, **e**). CT orbit shows bone lysis of superior orbital rim with associated soft tissue mass (**f**)

optic nerve can cause vision loss. Enophthalmos can also be a presentation of orbital tuberculosis due to the sclerosing effect of the mass lesion. Contiguous involvement of the brain parenchyma through superior orbital fissure can cause vision loss and other complications.

Tubercular involvement of orbital soft tissue can occur with or without orbital bone involvement. Periostitis and bony tuberculosis are the most common manifestations of orbital tuberculosis and is seen more commonly in children and young adults with average age of presentation being 8–14 years. The superior and lateral orbital walls are most commonly involved, and common clinical presentations include discharging sinus, proptosis, ophthalmoplegia and palpable orbital mass. Imaging reveals areas of bone lysis or sclerosis with or without associated soft tissue mass.

Paranasal sinus infection can involve the orbit by contiguous spread and presents as proptosis with orbital mass and globe displacement. The maxillary sinus is the most commonly involved, and history of nasal symptoms like epistaxis can be present in these patients. Tubercular dacryoadenitis is more common in adults and presents as lacrimal gland enlargement with or without associated pain.

Tubercular orbital infection is suspected based on the clinical and imaging findings and is confirmed by biopsy. According to Sen criteria, diagnosis is established by one or more of the following findings, (1) clinical, radiological or histopathological evidence of tuberculosis with a tubercular lesion elsewhere in the body, (2) positive culture and (3) AFB positivity [69]. Although open biopsy is required in most cases, FNAB from orbital mass can establish the diagnosis at times. Demonstration of the acid-fast bacilli on smear or culture of the *Mycobacterium tuberculosis* remains the gold standard for diagnosis. However, in cases where the bacillary load is low, like in extrapulmonary paucibacillary tuberculosis, culture and smear might give a false negative result. PCR for M tuberculosis has high specificity and can be used in some cases for confirmation of the diagnosis [70, 71]. However it has a low sensitivity. Ancillary investigations like chest X-ray and tuberculin skin test can be used along with the clinical evidence to confirm the diagnosis. The newer interferon-based immunological tests reduce the false positivity which is seen due to BCG vaccination and are highly specific unlike the tuberculin skin test [72, 73].

Antitubercular therapy remains the mainstay of treatment for orbital tuberculosis. DOTS (directly observed therapy, short course) regimen recommended by WHO uses four drugs for a duration of 6 months. The treatment regimen consists of initial four-drug therapy for 2 months (isoniazid, rifampicin, ethambutol, pyrazinamide) followed by 4 months of continuation phase with rifampicin and isoniazid. Ethambutol can cause optic neuropathy and is usually avoided in children where reliable visual assessment might not be possible. For extrapulmonary tuberculosis like orbital bone tuberculosis, an extended therapy might be needed. Surgery for orbital tuberculosis is indicated for diagnostic or therapeutic purposes as in cases of bone involvement with fistulae formation. Prognosis of orbital tuberculosis is usually favourable. Visual impairment due to optic atrophy has been reported in few cases; however, mortality due to orbital tuberculosis is rare.

Conclusion

Orbital infections are a common cause of proptosis. A thorough history to determine the aetiology and predisposing factors, systemic evaluation, imaging where appropriate, confirmation of the microbiological profile and determination of drug sensitivity, initiation of appropriate treatment along with supportive care and surgery where required can help resolve the condition with minimal morbidity and functional impairment.

Compliance with Ethical Requirements Sima Das and Santosh G. Honavar declare that they have no conflict of interest. No human studies were carried out by the authors for this article.

References

1. Van Dyke RB, Desky AB, Daum RS. Infections of the eye and periorbital structures. Adv Pediatr Infect Dis. 1988;3:125–79.
2. Ferguson MP, McNab AA. Current treatment and outcome in orbital cellulitis. Aust N Z J Ophthalmol. 1999;27(6):375–9.
3. Rubinstein JB, Handler SD. Orbital and periorbital cellulitis in children. Head Neck Surg. 1982;5(1):15–21.
4. Lessner A, Stern GA. Preseptal and orbital cellulitis. Infect Dis Clin North Am. 1992;6(4):933–52. Review.
5. Wald ER. Periorbital and orbital infections. Infect Dis Clin North Am. 2007;21(2):393–408. vi. Review.
6. Chandler JR, Langenbrunner DJ, Stevens ER. The pathogenesis of orbital complications in acute sinusitis. Laryngoscope. 1970;80(9):1414–28.
7. Philip J, Sylvester K. Post-traumatic orbital cellulitis. Br J Oral Maxillofac Surg. 2010;48(4):326.
8. Babar TF, Zaman M, Khan MN, Khan MD. Risk factors of preseptal and orbital cellulitis. J Coll Physicians Surg Pak. 2009;19(1):39–42.
9. Rimon A, Hoffer V, Prais D, Harel L, Amir J. Periorbital cellulitis in the era of Haemophilus influenzae type B vaccine: predisposing factors and etiologic agents in hospitalized children. J Pediatr Ophthalmol Strabismus. 2008;45(5):300–4.
10. McKinley SH, Yen MT, Miller AM, Yen KG. Microbiology of pediatric orbital cellulitis. Am J Ophthalmol. 2007;144(4):497–501.
11. Barone SR, Aiuto LT. Periorbital and orbital cellulitis in the Haemophilus influenzae vaccine era. J Pediatr Ophthalmol Strabismus. 1997;34(5):293–6.
12. Ambati BK, Ambati J, Azar N, Stratton L, Schmidt EV. Periorbital and orbital cellulitis before and after the advent of Haemophilus influenzae type B vaccination. Ophthalmology. 2000;107:1450–3.
13. Donahue SP, Schwartz G. Preseptal and orbital cellulitis in childhood. A changing microbiologic spectrum. Ophthalmology. 1998;105(10):1902–5; discussion 1905–6.
14. Vaska VL, Grimwood K, Gole GA, Nimmo GR, Paterson DL, Nissen MD. Community-associated methicillin-resistant Staphylococcus aureus causing orbital cellulitis in Australian children. Pediatr Infect Dis J. 2011;30(11):1003–6.
15. Argelich R, Ibáñez-Flores N, Bardavio J, Burés-Jelstrup A, García-Segarra G, Coll-Colell R, Cuadrado V, Fernández-Monrás F. Orbital cellulitis and endogenous endophthalmitis secondary to Proteus mirabilis cholecystitis. Diagn Microbiol Infect Dis. 2009; 64(4):442–4.
16. Luemsamran P, Pornpanich K, Vangveeravong S, Mekanandha P. Orbital cellulitis and endophthalmitis in pseudomonas septicemia. Orbit. 2008;27(6):455–7.
17. Peker E, Cagan E, Dogan M, Kilic A, Caksen H, Yesilmen O. Periorbital cellulitis caused by Bacillus thuringiensis. Eur J Ophthalmol. 2010;20(1):243–5.
18. Limjoco-Antonio AD, Janda WM, Schreckenberger PC. Arcanobacterium haemolyticum sinusitis and orbital cellulitis. Pediatr Infect Dis J. 2003;22(5):465–7.
19. Connell PP, Carey B, Kollpiara D, Fenton S. Kingella kingae orbital cellulitis in a 3-year-old. Eye (Lond). 2006;20(9):1086–8.
20. Mills DM, Meyer DR. Posttraumatic cellulitis and ulcerative conjunctivitis caused by Yersinia enterocolitica O:8. Ophthal Plast Reconstr Surg. 2008;24(5):425–6.
21. Smith AT, Spencer JT. Orbital complications resulting from lesions of the sinuses. Ann Otol Rhinol Laryngol. 1948;57(1):5–27.

22. Chandler JR, Langenbrunner DJ, Stevens ERL. The pathogenesis of orbital complications in acute sinusitis. Laryngoscope. 1970;80(9):1414–28.

23. Pandian DG, Babu RK, Chaitra A, Anjali A, Rao VA, Srinivasan R. Nine years' review on preseptal and orbital cellulitis and emergence of community-acquired methicillin-resistant Staphylococcus aureus in a tertiary hospital in India. Indian J Ophthalmol. 2011;59(6):431–5.

24. Robbins JB, Schneerson R, Arguman M, Hnadzel ZT. Haemophilus influenzae type b: disease and immunity in humans. Ann Intern Med. 1973;78(2): 259–69.

25. Kim IK, Kim JR, Jang KS, Moon YS, Park SW. Orbital abscess from an odontogenic infection. Oral Surg Oral Med Oral Pathol Oral Radiol Endod. 2007;103(1): e1–6. Epub 2006 Oct 6.

26. Colapinto P, Aslam SA, Frangouli O, Joshi N. Undiagnosed type 2 diabetes mellitus presenting with orbital cellulitis. Orbit 2008;27(5):380–2.

27. Ketenci I, Unlü Y, Vural A, Doğan H, Sahin MI, Tuncer E. Approaches to subperiosteal orbital abscesses. Eur Arch Otorhinolaryngol. 2013;270(4): 1317–27.

28. Sciarretta V, Macrì G, Farneti P, Tenti G, Bordonaro C, Pasquini E. Endoscopic surgery for the treatment of pediatric subperiosteal orbital abscess: a report of 10 cases. Int J Pediatr Otorhinolaryngol. 2009;73(12): 1669–72.

29. Todman MS, Enzer YR. Medical management versus surgical intervention of pediatric orbital cellulitis: the importance of subperiosteal abscess volume as a new criterion. Ophthal Plast Reconstr Surg. 2011;27: 255–9.

30. Kirszrot J, Rubin PA. Invasive fungal infections of the orbit. Int Ophthalmol Clin. 2007;47(2):117–32.

31. Klotz SA, Penn CC, Negvesky GJ, Butrus SI. Fungal and parasitic infections of the eye. Clin Microbiol Rev. 2000;13(4):662–85.

32. Brown J. Zygomycosis: an emerging fungal infection. Am J Health Syst Pharm. 2005;62(24):2593–6.

33. Wu VC, Wang R, Lai TS, Wu KD. Deferoxamine-related fatal nasal-orbital-cerebral mucormycosis. Kidney Int. 2006;70(11):1888.

34. Munir N, Jones NS. Rhinocerebral mucormycosis with orbital and intracranial extension: a case report and review of optimum management. J Laryngol Otol. 2007;121(2):192–5.

35. Spellberg B, Edwards Jr J, Ibrahim A. Novel perspectives on mucormycosis: pathophysiology, presentation, and management. Clin Microbiol Rev. 2005; 18(3):556–69.

36. Vehreschild JJ, Birtel A, Vehreschild MJ, Liss B, Farowski F, Kochanek M, Sieniawski M, Steinbach A, Wahlers K, Fätkenheuer G, Cornely OA. Mucormycosis treated with posaconazole: review of 96 case reports. Crit Rev Microbiol. 2013;39:310–24.

37. Seiff SR, Choo PH, Carter SR. Role of local amphotericin B therapy for sino-orbital fungal infections. Ophthal Plast Reconstr Surg. 1999;15(1):28–31.

38. Segal E, Menhusen MJ, Shawn S. Hyperbaric oxygen in the treatment of invasive fungal infections: a single-center experience. Isr Med Assoc J. 2007;9(5):355–7.

39. Levin LA, Avery R, Shore JW, Woog JJ, Baker AS. The spectrum of orbital aspergillosis: a clinicopathological review. Surv Ophthalmol. 1996;41(2):142–54.

40. DelGaudio JM, Swain Jr RE, Kingdom TT, Muller S, Hudgins PA. Computed tomographic findings in patients with invasive fungal sinusitis. Arch Otolaryngol Head Neck Surg. 2003;129(2):236–40.

41. Dhiwakar M, Thakar A, Bahadur S. Invasive sino-orbital aspergillosis: surgical decisions and dilemmas. J Laryngol Otol. 2003;117(4):280–5.

42. Arakawa H, Suto C, Notani H, Ishida T, Abe K, Ookubo Y. Selection of the antifungal agent decides prognosis of invasive aspergillosis: case report of a successful outcome with voriconazole. Int Ophthalmol. 2014; 34:85–9.

43. Mais FA. Cryosurgery in ocular cysticercosis [in Portuguese]. Rev Bras Oftalmol. 1969;28:99–106.

44. Malik SK, Gupta AK, Choudhry S. Ocular cysticercosis. Am J Ophthalmol. 1968;66:1168–71.

45. Sekhar GC, Honavar SG. Myocysticercosis: experience with imaging and therapy. Ophthalmology. 1999;106(12):2336–40.

46. Rath S, Honavar SG, Naik M, Anand R, Agarwal B, Krishnaiah S, Sekhar GC. Orbital cysticercosis: clinical manifestations, diagnosis, management, and outcome. Ophthalmology. 2010;117(3):600–5.

47. Malhotra R, Garg P, Mishra R, Khanduri S. Orbital cysticercosis: masquerading as orbital inflammatory disorder. Trop Doct. 2011;41(2):119–20.

48. El Hamdaoui M, Touitou V, Lehoang P. Orbital cysticercosis mimicking a painful third nerve palsy. J Fr Ophtalmol. 2012;35(10):818.e1–4.

49. Pushker N, Bajaj MS, Betharia SM. Orbital and adnexal cysticercosis. Clin Experiment Ophthalmol. 2002;30(5):322–33.

50. Singh U, Gupta P, Bansal R. Unusual presentation of orbital cysticercosis in subperiosteal space. J Pediatr Ophthalmol Strabismus. 2008;45(6):379–80.

51. Kaur A, Chaurasia S, Agrawal A. Cysticercosis of the bony orbit–a rare entity. Orbit. 2007;26(2):141–3.

52. Sen DK. Acute suppurative dacryoadenitis caused by a cysticercus cellulosa. J Pediatr Ophthalmol Strabismus. 1982;19(2):100–2.

53. Rosas N, Sotelo J, Nieto D. ELISA in the diagnosis of neurocysticercosis. Arch Neurol. 1986;43(4):353–6.

54. Honavar SG, Sekhar CG. Ultrasonological characteristics of extraocular cysticercosis. Orbit. 1998;17(4):271–84.

55. Sihota R, Honavar SG. Oral albendazole in the management of extraocular cysticercosis. Br J Ophthalmol. 1994;78(8):621–3.

56. McMannus DP, Zhang W, Bartley PB. Echinococcosis. Lancet. 2003;362:1295–304.

57. Khuroo MS. Hydatid disease: current status and recent advances. Ann Saudi Med. 2002;22:56–64.

58. King CH. Cestodes (tape worms). In: Mandell GL, Bennett JE, Dolin R, editors. Mandell, Douglas and Bennett'S, principles and practice of infectious

diseases. 6th ed. Philadelphia: Churchill Livingstone; 2005. pp. 3285–93.

59. Mahesh L, Biswas J, Subramanian N. Role of ultrasound and CT- scan in diagnosis of hydatid cyst of the orbit. Orbit. 2000;19:179–88.

60. Morales AG, Croxatto JO, Crovetto L, Ebner R. Hydatid cysts of the orbit, A review of 35 cases. Ophthalmology. 1998;95:1027–32.

61. Talib H. Orbital hydatid disease in Iraq. Br J Surg. 1972;59:391–4.

62. Murthy R, Honavar SG, Vemuganti GK, Naik M, Burman S. Polycystic echinococcosis of the orbit. Am J Ophthalmol. 2005;140(3):561–3.

63. Bagheri A, Fallahi MR, Yazdani S, Rezaee Kanavi M. Two different presentations of orbital echinococcosis: a report of two cases and review of the literature. Orbit. 2010;29(1):51–6.

64. Xiao A, Xueyi C. Hydatid cysts of the orbit in xinjiang: a review of 18 cases. Orbit. 1999;18:151–5.

65. Sihota R, Sharma T. Albendazole therapy for a recurrent orbital hydatid cyst. Indian J Ophthalmol. 2000;48(2):142–3.

66. Jimenénez-Mejías ME, Alarcón-Cruz JC, Márquez-Rivas FJ, Palomino-Nicás J, Montero JM, Pachón J. Orbital hydatid cyst: treatment and prevention of recurrences with albendazole plus praziquantel. J Infect. 2000;41(1):105–7.

67. Akhan O, Bilgiç S, Akata D, Kiratli H, Ozmen MN. Percutaneous treatment of an orbital hydatid cyst: a new therapeutic approach. Am J Ophthalmol. 1998;125(6):877–9.

68. Madge SN, Prabhakaran VC, Shome D, Kim U, Honavar S, Selva D. Orbital tuberculosis: a review of the literature. Orbit. 2008;27(4):267–77.

69. Sen DK. Tuberculosis of the orbit and lacrimal gland: a clinical study of 14 cases. J Pediatr Ophthalmol Strabismus. 1980;17:232–8.

70. Butt T, Ahmad RN, Kazmi SY, et al. An update on the diagnosis of tuberculosis. J Coll Physicians Surg Pak. 2003;13(12):728–34.

71. Cheng VCC, Yew WW, Yuen KY. Molecular diagnostics in tuberculosis. Eur J Clin Microbiol Infect Dis. 2005;24:711–20.

72. Connell TG, Rangaka MX, Curtis N, Wilkinson RJ. QuantiFERON-TB Gold: state of the art for the diagnosis of tuberculosis infection? Expert Rev Mol Diagn. 2006;6(5):663–77.

73. Nahid P, Madhukar P, Hopewell PC. Advances in the diagnosis and treatment of tuberculosis. Proc Am Thorac Soc. 2006;3:103–10.

Idiopathic Orbital Inflammation

2

Hakan Demirci

2.1 Background

Idiopathic orbital inflammation is a noninfectious, inflammatory process of the extraocular orbit and adnexa without underlying local or systemic etiology. It is a diagnosis of exclusion after neoplasm, infection, and systemic inflammatory disorders have been ruled out. It was first described by Gleason in 1903 and characterized as a distinct entity with the name of orbital pseudotumor by Birch-Hirschfeld in 1905 [1, 2]. Over the years, besides orbital pseudotumor other names such as nonspecific orbital inflammation, orbital inflammatory pseudotumor, and orbital inflammatory syndrome have also been used.

Depending on the origin of the study, idiopathic orbital inflammation constitutes 5–18 % of all orbital space-occupying lesions [3–5]. A review of 1,795 consecutive orbital tumors from Mayo Clinic showed that 8 % of all orbital tumors were inflammatory [6]. It was the third common orbital tumor followed by carcinoma and lymphoid tumors [6]. Similarly, in a review of 1,264 orbital tumors and simulating lesions that presented to Wills Eye Hospital over a

30-year period, 11 % of tumors were inflammatory lesions [3]. It was the second most common orbital lesion followed by lymphoid tumor.

2.2 Clinical Features

Idiopathic orbital inflammation mostly involves middle-aged people although it can affect any race, age, and sex. The only exception is that myositis and trochleitis, subtypes of idiopathic orbital inflammation, were found to be more common in females [7–10]. Pediatric cases make up 6–17 % of all cases of idiopathic orbital inflammation [4, 5]. Idiopathic orbital inflammation is usually a unilateral disease with almost equal involvement of the right and left orbits [11]. About a quarter of patients have bilateral disease [11]. A review of 209 patients from China showed that the mean age of the patients was 44 years (range 4–80 years). The right orbit was involved in 43 % of patients and the left orbit in 39 %, and both orbits were involved in 19 % of patients [12]. Clinical presentation of idiopathic orbital inflammation differs between children and adults. In children, bilateral involvement and associated systemic symptoms such as fever, malaise, lymphadenopathy, optic disk edema, uveitis, and tissue and peripheral blood eosinophilia are more common [13, 14]. Lacrimal gland enlargement or dacryoadenitis is the most common form of orbital inflammation in children [15].

H. Demirci, MD
Department of Ophthalmology and Visual Sciences,
W.K. Kellogg Eye Center, University of Michigan,
Ann Arbor, MI, USA
e-mail: hdemirci@umich.edu

H. Demirci (ed.), *Orbital Inflammatory Diseases and Their Differential Diagnosis*,
Essentials in Ophthalmology, DOI 10.1007/978-3-662-46528-8_2,
© Springer-Verlag Berlin Heidelberg 2015

Idiopathic orbital inflammation can have acute, subacute, or chronic presentation based on the onset and duration of symptoms [16]. Although presenting signs may change depending on the involved orbital structure(s), patients often present with periocular pain, periorbital edema and erythema, conjunctival injection, chemosis, proptosis, ptosis, diplopia, and pain with eye movements [16–19]. Pain is the most common symptom seen in 58–69 % of patients, followed by diplopia in 31–38 % of patients [4, 20]. Periorbital swelling is the most common sign seen in 75–79 % of patients, followed by proptosis in 32–63 %, restriction in extraocular motility in 54 %, conjunctival hyperemia in 48 %, chemosis in 29 %, decreased vision in 21 %, and ptosis in 17 % of patients [4, 20]. So, the patients with idiopathic orbital inflammation should evaluate a detailed eye examination, including visual acuity, orbital and external eye examinations, slit lamp examination, and detailed eye examination.

Patients with acute presentation have predominantly inflammatory signs such as pain, periorbital edema, and erythema. Patients with subacute and chronic presentation have predominantly mass effect such as proptosis, limitation in extraocular motility, and vertical globe displacement. The amount of proptosis might change according to the degree of inflammation, fibrosis, and mass effect. Idiopathic orbital inflammation can affect the orbit, as local, encapsulated mass or diffuse inflammation, or any tissue in the orbit including the lacrimal gland, extraocular muscle, sclera, or trochlea or around the optic nerve. In Tolosa-Hunt syndrome or orbital apex syndrome when the inflammation involves the orbital apex as well as cavernous sinus and superior orbital fissure, patients present with severe, unilateral headache with extraocular palsies, involving the third, fourth, fifth, and sixth cranial nerves. A review of 132 patients with idiopathic orbital inflammation showed that diffuse inflammatory process was the most frequent presentation in 40 patients (30 %) followed by myositis in 21 patients (16 %), dacryoadenitis in 14 patients (11 %), focal encapsulated inflammatory process in 5 patients (4 %), Tolosa-Hunt syndrome in 2 patients (2 %), perineuritis in 1 patient (1 %), and scleritis in 1 patient

(1 %) [21]. Extraorbital extension of inflammation is rare but has been reported to occur into the intracranial cavity, paranasal sinuses, and pterygopalatine fossa and is best evaluated with an imaging study like computed tomography or magnetic resonance imaging [21–29].

2.3　Classification

Several classifications have been used for idiopathic orbital inflammation based on the onset of inflammation, involved orbital structures, and pathologic features [30]. Idiopathic orbital inflammation is classified into acute, subacute, and chronic forms based on the onset of the inflammation [30]. If the onset of symptoms is less than 2 weeks, it is classified as acute idiopathic orbital inflammation. If it is between 2 and 4 weeks, it is subacute idiopathic orbital inflammation, and if it is more than 4 weeks, then it is chronic idiopathic orbital inflammation. Idiopathic orbital inflammation is classified as dacryoadenitis when it involved the lacrimal gland, myositis when it involved the extraocular muscle or muscles, scleritis when it involved the sclera, optic neuritis when it involved the optic nerve, Tolosa-Hunt syndrome when it involved the superior orbital fissure, and cavernous sinus or diffuse orbital inflammation when it diffusely involved the orbital tissue [30]. Depending on the pathologic features, it is classified as predominantly lymphoid, granulomatous, sclerosing, eosinophilic, and vasculitic inflammation [30]. Bijlsma et al. [31] evaluated the classification systems of IOI in 84 patients and concluded that classification systems based on histopathology and localization showed good reliability, were easy to apply, and described the biologic process.

2.4　Pathophysiology

The etiology and pathogenesis of idiopathic orbital inflammation is unknown. Orbital myositis and dacryoadenitis have been reported to start simultaneously or within several weeks of streptococcal pharyngitis, Lyme disease, and herpes zoster ophthalmicus in several case reports [32–35]. Mollicutes are cell wall-deficient bacteria and found in cases with chronic uveitis. Wirostko et al. [36] proposed that parasitizing followed by destruction of orbital leukocytes by mollicute-like organisms led to vasculitis, tissue lysis, lymphoid infiltrates, and granuloma formation.

Orbital inflammation has been observed in rheumatologic conditions like Crohn's disease, systemic lupus erythematous, rheumatoid arthritis, myasthenia gravis, and ankylosing spondylitis. In a series of idiopathic orbital inflammation and refractory ocular inflammation, coinciding rheumatologic or autoimmune disease has been present between 10 and 78 % of cases [37, 38]. Similarly, circulating autoantibodies against eye muscle membrane proteins of 55 and 64 kilodaltons were seen in 63 % of orbital myositis patients compared to 16–20 % of healthy people [39]. However, unilateral presentation and limited muscle involvement argue against the role of circulating autoantibodies in idiopathic orbital inflammation. Mottow-Lippe et al. [14] suggested that the release of circulating antigens caused by local vascular permeability triggered an inflammatory response in the orbit. They proposed that the network of connective tissue and capillaries in the orbit played a role in delivering antigenic agents to different orbital structures and hence different clinical presentations.

Studies evaluating molecular biologic environment of idiopathic orbital inflammation showed that interleukin-2, interleukin-8, interleukin-10, interleukin-12, gamma interferon, and tumor necrosis factor alpha were significantly elevated in the orbital tissue of idiopathic orbital inflammation patients compared to normal orbital tissue [40]. Among these, gamma interferon and interleukin-12 were expressed ten times higher concentrations than normal controls. Interleukin-12, produced by antigen-producing cells, promotes the production of Th1 cells and induces the production of interferon gamma, the chief product of Th1 cells. TNF-alpha is a critical mediator of induction of Th1 response. These suggest that Th1 pathway plays an important role in the pathogenesis of idiopathic orbital inflammation. Later, same authors reported that

Toll-like receptors (TLR) especially TLR2 were markedly expressed in idiopathic orbital inflammation [41]. TLRs are receptors that are usually expressed in macrophages and dendritic cells, which are part of the innate immune system.

2.5   Diagnosis

By definition, idiopathic orbital inflammation is a diagnosis of exclusion. The patients with idiopathic orbital inflammation need systemic evaluation to exclude the other local and systemic causes of orbital inflammation. In the history, the presence of similar previous episodes, trauma, infection, systemic or immunocompromised conditions, and duration of symptoms need to be evaluated. As a part of systemic work-up, imaging of the orbit with computed tomography or magnetic resonance imaging, chest X-ray, complete blood count, angiotensin-converting enzyme and lysozyme levels, cytoplasmic and perinuclear antineutrophil cytoplasmic antibody, rapid plasma regain test, and thyroid function studies – T3, T4, thyroid-stimulating hormone, thyroid-stimulating immunoglobulin, and thyrotropin receptor antibody – should be ordered [4].

Computed imaging (CT) is the first choice of orbital imaging. On CT, idiopathic orbital inflammation shows diffuse homogenous involvement of the orbital soft tissue or homogenous enlargement of the involved orbital tissue such as the extraocular muscles, lacrimal gland, sclera, optic nerve sheath, or trochlea. The involved tissue demonstrates enhancement with contrast in computed tomography and has irregular borders. CT features might change from subtle infiltrative changes affecting specific orbital structures to almost complete orbit involvement [42]. There is usually no bony erosion, and if any bony erosion is seen, alternative etiologies should be in the differential diagnosis. Magnetic resonance imaging (MRI) and orbital ultrasonography may also be used as adjunct diagnostic imaging tools. On MRI, orbital inflammation appears as homogenous orbital mass that is isointense to extraocular muscles on T1- and T2-weighted images, while orbital cellulitis appears hyperintense to extraocular muscles [18]. There is homogenous enhancement of the involved tissue with gadolinium. Diffusion-weighted imaging of MRI showed significant difference in image intensity and apparent diffusion coefficients between orbital lymphoid lesions, orbital cellulitis, and idiopathic orbital inflammation [43]. Orbital lymphoid lesions were the brightest followed by idiopathic orbital inflammation and orbital cellulitis. Traditionally, homogenous enlargement of the extraocular muscle with tendon involvement on imaging studies has been used to differentiate idiopathic orbital inflammation from Graves' eye disease because the tendon is typically spared in Graves' eye disease [44]. However, occasional tendon involvement was reported in Graves' eye disease, especially in the patients with primary gaze diplopia [44]. Ultrasonography is helpful in the evaluation of swelling around the sclera and optic nerve that appears as a "T sign" in scleritis or at the tendon of extraocular muscles [18].

The diagnosis of idiopathic orbital inflammation is usually based on clinical and radiologic findings; however, biopsy is required to confirm the diagnosis histopathologically and to exclude other possible diseases. In the past, some authors proposed that biopsy was not required for the diagnosis of idiopathic orbital inflammation [45, 46]. The relief of signs and symptoms by systemic corticosteroids was used to confirm the initial clinical diagnosis. However, the clinical and radiologic features of idiopathic orbital inflammation are not specific. Orbital tumors such as lymphoma or orbital involvement in systemic inflammatory disorders may have similar clinical and radiologic features, and they can regress in response to systemic corticosteroid. The biopsy should be performed before any therapy, because any form of immunosuppressive treatment might change the histopathologic features, making the diagnosis difficult.

2.6   Histopathology

On histopathologic examination, idiopathic orbital inflammation shows an infiltrate of inflammatory cells mainly of small, well-differentiated mature lymphocytes, admixed with plasma cells, neutrophils, eosinophils, and occasionally macrophages and histiocytes [30, 47]. When infiltrated lymphocytes are assessed, T lymphocytes outnumber the B lymphocytes, and T-helper cells are predominant over T-suppressor cells [30, 48]. B and T lymphocytes are immunophenotypically polyclonal. On immunohistochemistry, orbital inflammation tissue showed strong expression of B-cell marker CD20 in 5–25 % of lymphocytes, moderate expression of another B-cell marker CD22 in 2–70 % of lymphocytes, strong expression of a B-cell and dendritic cell marker CD23 in 5 % of dendritic cells, strong expression of an interleukin-2 receptor marker CD25 found on the activated T and B cells in 10–60 % of lymphocytes, and moderate expression of T-cell marker CD3 in 60 % of lymphocytes [49].

Histopathologic features vary depending on the stages of inflammation. In acute stages of inflammation, lymphocytes, plasma cells, and eosinophils are more numerous, while with chronic disease, lymphocytes, plasma cells, and occasionally macrophages predominate with increasing fibrosis among cells and along the septa, radiating into the orbital fat [50]. There are always associated stromal changes, including edema in acute inflammation and proliferative fibrosis, sclerosis, and hyalinization in chronic inflammation. Previously, fibrosis/sclerosis was thought to be the result of severe and long-standing inflammation; however, the sclerosing form of idiopathic orbital inflammation showed that fibrosis is an immune-mediated process with fibrosis in early stages of inflammation [51]. The presence of eosinophils and its cytotoxic contents in the fibrosis areas suggest that they play a role in the formation of fibrosis [52]. Orbital fat is infiltrated by lymphocytes and plasma cells, appearing as a mixed inflammatory infiltrate with increased fibrous tissue, and the orbital septa are thickened because of the increased fibroblastic tissue. Lymphoid follicles with reactive germinal center can be seen in varying amounts. Perivasculitis or angiocentric lymphocytic cuffing is the most common vascular change due to concentration of lymphocytes, occasionally plasma cells and eosinophils in the immediate adventitial area of the capillaries and postcapillary venules [30, 50].

Histopathologically, subtypes of idiopathic orbital inflammation include lymphocytic, granulomatous, sclerosing, and vasculitic or eosinophilic. Granulomatous idiopathic orbital inflammation is rare and presents in a spectrum of histopathologic spectrum, including non-necrotizing foreign body type granulomas, lipogranulomatous inflammation and variable sclerosis [53, 54]. In idiopathic sclerosing orbital inflammation, sclerosis and hyalinization predominate with paucity of inflammatory cells consisting of predominantly T lymphocytes, few eosinophils, histiocytes, and plasma cells [51, 55]. It is a distinct clinical entity and represents about 8 % of all inflammatory lesions of the orbit [51]. Idiopathic sclerosing orbital inflammation might be associated with other fibrosclerosing disorders such as retroperitoneal fibrosis, Riedel's thyroiditis, mesenteritis, sclerosing cholangitis, and mediastinal fibrosis [48, 56–59]. It has a slow progression and may result in worse visual outcome due to response to conventional treatment [16, 60, 61]. It usually requires more aggressive and prolonged treatment [16, 55]. In these patients, an immunosuppressive agent might be needed in addition to the systemic corticosteroid. A review of the literature showed that 67 % of cases with idiopathic sclerosing orbital pseudotumor involved the anterior orbital and lacrimal gland, 56 % midorbit, and 51 % posterior orbit and extraocular muscles [55]. The most commonly involved quadrant was lateral and/or superior in 54 % of cases. Corticosteroid alone or in combination with other modalities was the most common choice of treatment. Treatment outcome for steroid alone was good in 43 % of cases, partial in 24 %, and poor in 33 % of cases. The overall response, regardless of treatment regimen, was good in 31 %, partial in 39 %, and poor in 21 % of cases.

When the lacrimal gland is involved, focal aggregates and follicles of lymphocytes and plasma cells are observed. Periductal and periacinar fibrosis, ductal dilatation, acinar atrophy, and thickened interlobular tissue septa separating the lobules are the features of lacrimal gland involvement. In myositis, the muscle fibers are swollen and infiltrated with lymphocytes and plasma cells in a diffuse or multifocal pattern and separated by edema and fibrosis.

2.7   Differential Diagnosis

The differential diagnosis of idiopathic orbital inflammation includes orbital cellulitis, Graves' eye disease, lymphoproliferative disorders, arteriovenous malformation and lymphangioma, metastatic carcinoma, retained foreign body, and ruptured dermoid cyst. Orbital cellulitis is usually associated with sinusitis, facial or eyelid infection, and trauma. Patients with orbital cellulitis present with fever, elevated white blood cell count, proptosis, chemosis, ptosis, and restriction of motility [62, 63]. Orbital imaging might show decreased orbital fat signal, concurrent sinus disease, bony erosion, and subperiosteal abscess. Graves' eye disease is an autoimmune inflammatory disorder that is commonly associated with hyperthyroidism but may occur in the euthyroid setting [64, 65]. It presents with eyelid retraction, eyelid lag, proptosis, restriction in motility, and compressive optic neuropathy. In contrast to the abrupt onset of pain and inflammatory signs in idiopathic orbital inflammation, Graves' eye disease usually has a slower, more insidious course. Graves' eye disease usually involves both orbits but can be asymmetric. The distinction between lymphoproliferative disorders and idiopathic orbital inflammation is based on clinical and mostly histopathologic findings. Clinically, lymphoproliferative disorders are seen in elder patients, have an insidious onset, and show slow progression. They are associated with symptoms and signs related to mass effect rather than inflammation [66]. Histopathologically, lymphoproliferative disorders demonstrate a homogenous monoclonal lymphocyte cell population with high lambda-kappa ratio. Other disorders that may be accompanied by a significant inflammatory reaction and present similar clinical picture include orbital arteriovenous malformation, lymphangioma, and ruptured dermoid cysts. Orbital imaging might be helpful in differentiation of these problems. A history of orbital trauma and potential retained intraorbital foreign body causing inflammation should also be investigated. Metastatic orbital tumors, primary ocular tumors with extrascleral extension such as uveal melanoma, or necrotic retinoblastoma might present with similar clinical pictures and should be excluded.

2.8   Treatment of Idiopathic Orbital Inflammation

Management of idiopathic orbital inflammation includes observation, nonsteroidal anti-inflammatory agents, corticosteroids, immuno-suppressive agents, immunotherapy, and external beam radiotherapy. Asymptomatic cases with mild inflammation and in whom vision was not threatened might be observed. In their review of 24 cases with idiopathic orbital inflammation, Swamy et al. [47] reported that 21 % of them were observed without any therapy and did not have any recurrence after a median of 23 months of follow-up. Nonsteroidal anti-inflammatory therapy has been used in the management of idiopathic orbital inflammation, especially for orbital myositis. Manor et al. [67] suggested to treat orbital myositis initially with a nonsteroidal anti-inflammatory therapy and observed that 65 % of their cases responded to this therapy without any recurrence. They used systemic corticosteroid therapy for cases refractory to this therapy.

Systemic corticosteroids are the main therapy for idiopathic orbital inflammation. They usually produce rapid and dramatic improvement of signs and symptoms. In an earlier study, Mombaerts et al. [68] reported that 78 % of patients with idiopathic orbital inflammation had a positive initial response to systemic corticosteroids, but only 37 % of them were cured and 52 % showed recurrence. While 95 % of patients with optic neuropathy recovered following systemic corticosteroids, patients with sclerosing and vasculitis subtype had a poor response. Yuen and Rubin [4] reported that 47 % of patients with idiopathic orbital inflammation showed treatment success with systemic corticosteroids,

33 % developed steroid dependence, and 13 % had steroid intolerance. Systemic steroids can be administered orally or pulsed intravenously. In non-vision threatening cases and those without optic nerve compression, oral steroids are initiated. The typical starting dose is between 1–1.5 mg/kg and 60–100 mg of oral prednisone, and a slow taper is recommended over weeks to months to prevent recurrence [69]. Intravenous treatment can be used in atypical cases, those with associated vision loss, or in cases refractory to oral administration [70]. Recurrent disease during or after steroid taper is common in adults, though rarely reported in the pediatric population [14]. When intravenous methylprednisolone plus oral prednisone with oral prednisone alone was compared in the treatment of idiopathic orbital inflammation, no difference in duration of therapy, symptom-free outcome, or recurrence rate was noted [71]. The only difference was the faster symptom relief and recovery from optic nerve symptoms. Localized intraorbital injection of corticosteroids has been used in the management of idiopathic orbital inflammation [70]. Localized intraorbital injection has been reported to have efficacy in patients with anterior idiopathic orbital inflammation and in a case of biopsy-proven idiopathic orbital inflammation unresponsive to systemic steroid administration [72, 73]. In addition, it may be used in children or diabetics to reduce the systemic side effects of corticosteroid use.

External beam radiotherapy has been used for patients who are resistant or intolerant to systemic corticosteroid therapy. Radiation dose varying from 1,000 to 3,000 cGy over 10–15 days has been used in the treatment of idiopathic orbital inflammation [74–76]. A review of 24 patients showed improvement in 87 % of patients with soft tissue swelling, in 82 % of patients with proptosis, in 78 % of patients with restriction of extraocular motility, and in 75 % of patients with pain [77]. Response to external beam radiotherapy varies depending on the subtype of idiopathic orbital inflammation. The patients with myositis variant respond well to external beam radiotherapy, while patients with sclerosing or granulomatous variant have a poor response, and patients with the vasculitis variant show variable response [51, 68, 78, 79].

The use of steroid-sparing agents including antimetabolites, T-cell inhibitors, and alkylating agents has been reported in patients who are not responsive to steroid treatment, have a chronic progressive course, and require long-term immunosuppression or in combination with steroids as first-line treatment in patients with idiopathic sclerosing inflammation [22, 80–82]. Medications that have been used in idiopathic orbital inflammation patients include methotrexate, azathioprine, mycophenolate mofetil, cyclophosphamide, tacrolimus, and cyclosporine [80, 82–85]. Among these agents, methotrexate is a commonly used one. It has been used 15–25 mg/week for the duration of ranging from 4 to 34 weeks. It has been reported that 57–73 % of patients showed reduction of inflammatory activity. In a review of 22 patients who used low dose of 12.5 mg/week systemic corticosteroid therapy, Shah et al. [85] observed that 64 % of patients were able to taper or discontinue corticosteroid therapy and 23 % of patients showed complete remission. Biologic agents like monoclonal antibody against tumor necrosis factor alpha and CD20 receptors have been used in the treatment of idiopathic orbital inflammation. There are case reports that show response to adalimumab, daclizumab, and rituximab therapy. Garrity et al. [38] reported favorable response in all seven patients with chronic and refractory orbital myositis after a dosing schedule of 3–5 mg/kg given at weeks 0, 2, and 6 with treatments every 4–8 weeks afterward.

Surgical debulking is rarely performed, but may have a role in the treatment of sclerosing forms of idiopathic orbital inflammation with significant mass effect, fibrosis, and scarring. Orbital exenteration may be indicated in select cases where diffuse orbital involvement results in vision loss and pain unresponsive to other medical or radiation therapy [4].

Compliance with Ethical Requirements Hakan Demirci declares that he has no conflict of interest.

No human or animal studies were carried out by the authors for this article.

References

1. Gleason JE. Idiopathic myositis involving the extraocular muscles. Ophthalmic Rec. 1903;12:471–8.
2. Birch-Hirschfeld A. Zur diagnostic and pathologic der orbital tumoren. Ber zusammenkunft Dtsch Ophthalmol Ges. 1905;32:127–35.
3. Shields JA, Shields CL, Scartozzi R. Survey of 1264 patients with orbital tumors and simulating lesions: The 2002 Montgomery Lecture, part 1. Ophthalmology. 2004;111:997–1008.
4. Yuen SJ, Rubin PA. Idiopathic orbital inflammation. Distribution, clinical features and treatment outcome. Arch Ophthalmol. 2003;121:491–9.
5. Rubin PA, Foster CS. Etiology and management of idiopathic orbital inflammation. Am J Ophthalmol. 2004;138:1041–3.
6. Garrity JA, Henderson JW. The tumor surgery in the Henderson's orbital tumors. 4th ed. Philadelphia: Lippincott Williams & Wilkins; 2007. p. 23–32.
7. Gordon LK. Orbital inflammatory disease: a diagnostic and therapeutic challenge. Eye (London). 2006;20:1196–206.
8. Kitei D, DiMario Jr FJ. Childhood orbital pseudotumor: case report and literature review. J Child Neurol. 2008;23:425–30.
9. Scott IU, Siatkowski RM. Idiopathic orbital myositis. Curr Opin Rheumatol. 1997;9:504–12.
10. Siatkowski RM, Capo H, Byrne SF, et al. Clinical and echographic findings in idiopathic orbital myositis. Am J Ophthalmol. 1994;118:343–50.
11. Mendenhall WM, Lessner AM. Orbital pseudotumor. Am J Clin Oncol. 2010;33:304–6.
12. Yan J, Wu Z, Li Y. The differentiation of idiopathic inflammatory pseudotumor from lymphoid tumors of orbit: analysis of 319 cases. Orbit. 2004;23:245–54.
13. Berger JW, Rubin PA, Jakobiec FA. Pediatric orbital pseudotumor: case report and review of the literature. Int Ophthalmol Clin. 1996;36(1):161–77.
14. Mottow-Lippa L, Jakobiec FA, Smith M. Idiopathic inflammatory orbital pseudotumor in childhood II. Results of diagnostic tests and biopsies. Ophthalmology. 1981;88:565–74.
15. Belanger C, Zhang KS, Reddy AK, Yen MY, Yen KG. Inflammatory disorders of the orbit in childhood: a case series. Am J Ophthalmol. 2010;150:460–3.
16. Gupta S, Demirci H, Lee BJ, Elner VM, Kahana A, et al. Orbital inflammation. In: Smith and Nesi's ophthalmic plastic and reconstructive surgery. New York: Springer; 2012. pp.
17. Rootman J. Inflammatory diseases. In: Rootman J, editor. Diseases of the orbit: a multidisciplinary approach. 2nd ed. Philadelphia: Lippincott Williams & Wilkins; 2003. p. 455–506.
18. Cockerham KP, Hong SH, Browne EE. Orbital inflammation. Curr Neurol Neurosci Rep. 2003;3(5):401–9.
19. Weber AL, Jakobiec FA, Sabates NR. Pseudotumor of the orbit. Neuroimaging Clin N Am. 1996;6(1):73–92.
20. Chaudhry IA, Shamsi FA, Arat YO, Riley FC. Orbital pseudotumor: distinct diagnostic features and

management. Middle East Afr J Ophthalmol. 2008;15: 17–27.

21. Gunalp I, Gunduz K, Yazar Z. Idiopathic orbital inflammatory disease. Acta Ophthalmol Scand. 1996; 74:191–3.

22. Zborowska B, Ghabrial R, Selva D, McCluskey P. Idiopathic orbital inflammation with extraorbital extension: case series and review. Eye (London). 2006;20:107–13.

23. Tay E, Gibson A, Chaudhary N, Olver J. Idiopathic orbital inflammation with extensive intra- and extra-cranial extension presenting as 6th nerve palsy – a case report and literature review. Orbit. 2008;27:458–61.

24. de Jesus O, Inserni JA, Gonzalez A, Colon LE. Idiopathic orbital inflammation with intracranial extension. Case report. J Neurosurg. 1996;85:510–3.

25. Cruz AA, Akaishi PM, Chahud F, Elias JJ. Sclerosing inflammation in the orbit and in the pterygopalatine and infratemporal fossae. Ophthal Plast Reconstr Surg. 2003;19:201–6.

26. Kaye AH, Hahn JF, Craciun A, Hanson M, Berlin AJ, Tubbs RR. Intracranial extension of inflammatory pseudotumor of the orbit. Case report. J Neurosurg. 1984;60:625–9.

27. Bencherif B, Zouaoui A, Chedid G, Kujas M, Van Effenterre R, Marsault C. Intracranial extension of an idiopathic orbital inflammatory pseudotumor. AJNR Am J Neuroradiol. 1993;14:181–4.

28. Noble SC, Chandler WF, Lloyd RV. Intracranial extension of orbital pseudotumor: a case report. Neurosurgery. 1986;18:798–801.

29. Frohman LP, Kupersmith MJ, Lang J, et al. Intracranial extension and bone destruction in orbital pseudotu-mor. Arch Ophthalmol. 1986;104:380–4.

30. Mombaerts I, Goldschmeding R, Schlingemann RO, Koorneef L. What is orbital pseudotumor? Surv Ophthalmol. 1996;41:66–78.

31. Bijlsma WR, Vant Hullenaar FC, Mourits MP, Kalmann R. Evaluation of classification systems for nonspecific idiopathic orbital inflammation. Orbit. 2012;31:238–45.

32. Purcell JJ, Taulbee WA. Orbital myositis after upper respiratory tract infection. Arch Ophthalmol. 1981; 99:437–8.

33. Nieto JC, Kim N, Lucarelli MJ. Dacryoadenitis and orbital myositis associated with lyme disease. Arch Ophthalmol. 2008;126:1165–6.

34. Kawasaki A, Borruat FX. An unusual presentation of herpes zoster ophthalmicus: orbital myositis preceding vesicular eruption. Am J Ophthalmol. 2003;136:574–5.

35. Alshaikh M, Kakakios AM, Kemp AS. Orbital myosi-tis following streptococcal pharyngitis. J Paediatr Child Health. 2008;44:233–4.

36. Wirostko E, Johnson L, Wirostko B. Chronic orbital inflammatory disease: parasitisation of orbital leuko-cytes by mollicute-like organisms. Br J Ophthalmol. 1989;73:865–70.

37. Sobrin L, Kim E, Christen W, et al. Infliximab therapy for the treatment of refractory ocular inflammatory disease. Arch Ophthalmol. 2007;125:895–900.

38. Garrity JA, Coleman AW, Matteson EL, et al. Treatment of recalcitrant idiopathic orbital inflamma-tion (chronic orbital myositis) with infliximab. Am J Ophthalmol. 2004;138:925–30.

39. Atabay C, Tyutyunikov A, Scalise D, et al. Serum antibodies reactive with eye muscle membrane anti-gens are detected in patients with nonspecific orbital inflammation. Ophthalmology. 1995;102:145–53.

40. Wladis EJ, Iglesias BV, Gosselin EJ. Characterization of the molecular biologic milieu of idiopathic orbital inflammation. Ophthal Plast Reconstr Surg. 2011;27:251.

41. Wladis EJ, Iglesias BV, Adam AP, Nazeer T, Gosslein EJ. Toll-like receptors in idiopathic orbital inflamma-tion. Ophthal Plast Reconstr Surg. 2012;28:273–6.

42. De Wyngaert R, Casteels I, Demaerel P. Orbital and anterior visual pathway infection and inflammation. Neuroradiology. 2009;51:385–96.

43. Kapur R, Sepahdari AR, Mafee MF, et al. MR imag-ing of orbital inflammatory syndrome, orbital celluli-tis, and orbital lymphoid lesions: the role of diffusion-weighted imaging. AJNR Am J Neuroradiol. 2009;30:64–70.

44. Ben Simon GJ, Syed HM, Douglas R, McCann JD, Goldberg RA. Extraocular muscle enlargement with tendon involvement in thyroid-associated orbitopathy. Am J Ophthalmol. 2004;137:1145–7.

45. Mauriello Jr JA, Flanagan JC. Management of orbital inflammatory disease. A protocol. Surv Ophthalmol. 1984;29:104–16.

46. Kennerdell JS, Dresner SC. The nonspecific orbital inflam-matory syndromes. Surv Ophthalmol. 1984;29:93–103.

47. Swamy BN, McCluskey P, Nemet A, Crouch R, Martin P, Benger R, Ghabriel R, Wakefield D. Idiopathic orbital inflammatory syndrome: clinical features and treatment outcomes. Br J Ophthalmol. 2007;91:1667–70.

48. McCarthy JM, White VA, Harris G, et al. Idiopathic sclerosing inflammation of the orbit: immunohisto-logic analysis and comparison with retroperitoneal fibrosis. Mod Pathol. 1993;6:581–7.

49. Ho VH, Chevez-Barrios P, Jorgensen JL, Silkis RZ, Esmaeli B. Receptor expression in orbital inflamma-tory syndromes and implications for targeted therapy. Tissue Antigens. 2007;70:105–9.

50. Jakobiec FA, Font RL. Noninfectious orbital inflam-mations. In: Spence WH, editor. Ophthalmic pathol-ogy: an atlas and textbook, vol. 3. 3rd ed. Philadelphia: WB Saunders; 1986. p. 2777–95.

51. Rootman J, McCarthy M, White V, et al. Idiopathic scle-rosing inflammation of the orbit. A distinct clinicopath-ological entity. Ophthalmology. 1994;101:570–84.

52. Nogushi H, Kephart GM, Campbell J, et al. Tissue eosinophilia and eosinophil degranulation in orbital pseudotumor. Ophthalmology. 1991;98:928–32.

53. Raskin EM, McCormick S, Maher EA, Della Rocca RC. Granulomatous idiopathic orbital inflammation. Ophthal Plast Reconstr Surg. 1995;11:131–5.

54. Mombaerts I, Schlingemann RO, Gold.schmeding R, Koornneef L. Idiopathic granulomatous orbital inflammation. Ophthalmology. 1996;103:2135–41.

55. Pemberton JD, Fay A. Idiopathic sclerosing orbital inflammation: a review of demographics, clinical presentation, imaging, pathology, treatment, and outcome. Ophthal Plast Reconstr Surg. 2012;28:79–83.

56. Levine MR, Kaye L, Mair S, Bates J. Multifocal fibrosclerosis. Report of a case of bilateral idiopathic sclerosing pseudotumor and retroperitoneal fibrosis. Arch Ophthalmol. 1993;111:841–3.

57. Comings DE, Skubi KB, Van Eyes J, Motulsky AG. Familial multifocal fibrosclerosis. Findings suggesting that retroperitoneal fibrosis, mediastinal fibrosis, sclerosing cholangitis, Riedel's thyroiditis, and pseudotumor of the orbit may be different manifestations of a single disease. Ann Intern Med. 1967;66: 884–92.

58. Egsgaard Nielsen V, Hecht P, Krogdahl AS, et al. A rare case of orbital involvement in Riedel's thyroiditis. J Endocrinol Invest. 2003;26:1032–6.

59. Schaffler GJ, Simbrunner J, Lechner H, et al. Idiopathic sclerotic inflammation of the orbit with left optic nerve compression in a patient with multifocal fibrosclerosis. AJNR Am J Neuroradiol. 2000;21:194–7.

60. Hsuan JD, Selva D, McNab AA, Sullivan TJ, Saeed P, O'Donnell BA. Idiopathic sclerosing orbital inflammation. Arch Ophthalmol. 2006;124:1244–50.

61. Chen YM, Hu FR, Liao SL. Idiopathic sclerosing orbital inflammation – a case series study. Ophthalmologica. 2010;224:55–8.

62. Espinoza GM. Orbital inflammatory pseudotumors: etiology, differential diagnosis, and management. Curr Rheumatol Rep. 2010;12:443–7.

63. Mawn LA, Jordan DR, Donahue SP. Preseptal and orbital cellulitis. Ophthalmol Clin North Am. 2000;13:633–41.

64. Cockerham KP, Chan SS. Thyroid eye disease. Neurol Clin. 2010;28:729–55.

65. Briceno CA, Guspta S, Douglas RS. Advances in the management of thyroid eye disease. Int Ophthalmol Clin. 2013;53:93–101.

66. Watkins LM, Carter KD, Nerad JA. Ocular adnexal lymphoma of the extraocular muscles: case series from the University of Iowa and review of the literature. Ophthal Plast Reconstr Surg. 2011;27:471–6.

67. Mannor GE, Rose GE, Moseley IF, Wright JE. Outcome of orbital myositis. Clinical features associated with recurrence. Ophthalmology. 1997;104:409–13.

68. Mombaerts I, Schlingemann RO, Goldschmeding R, Koornneef L. Are systemic corticosteroids useful in the management of orbital pseudotumors? Ophthalmology. 1996;103:521–8.

69. Jacobs D, Galetta S. Diagnosis and management of orbital pseudo- tumor. Curr Opin Ophthalmol. 2002;13(6):347–51.

70. Harris GJ. Idiopathic orbital inflammation: a pathogenetic construct and treatment strategy: the 2005 ASOPRS foundation lecture. Ophthal Plast Reconstr Surg. 2006;22:79–86.

71. Bijlsma WR, Paridaens D, Kalmann R. Treatment of severe idiopathic orbital inflammation with intravenous methylprednisolone. Br J Ophthalmol. 2011;95: 1068–71.

72. Leibovitch I, Prabhakaran VC, Davis G, Selva D. Intraorbital injection of triamcinolone acetonide in patients with idiopathic orbital inflammation. Arch Ophthalmol. 2007;125:1647–51.

73. Skaat A, Rosen N, Rosner M, Schiby G, Simon GJ. Triamcinolone acetonide injection for persistent atypical idiopathic orbital inflammation. Orbit. 2009; 28:401–3.

74. Orcutt J, Garner A, Henk J, Wright J. Treatment of idiopathic inflammatory orbital pseudotumors by radiotherapy. Br J Ophthalmol. 1983;67:570–4.

75. Kennerdell J, Johnson B, Deutsch M. Radiation treatment of orbital lymphoid hyperplasia. Ophthalmology. 1979;86:942–7.

76. Sergott R, Glaser J, Charyulu K. Radiotherapy for idiopathic inflammatory orbital pseudotumor: indications and results. Arch Ophthalmol. 1981;99:8536.

77. Lanciano R, Fowble B, Sergoot RC, et al. The results of radiotherapy for orbital pseudotumor. Int J Radiat Oncol Biol Phys. 1990;18:407–11.

78. Snebold NG. Orbital pseudotumor syndromes. Curr Opin Ophthalmol. 1997;8:41–4.

79. Garrity JA, Kennerdell JS, Johnson B, et al. Cyclophosphamide in the treatment of orbital vasculitis. Am J Ophthalmol. 1986;102:97–103.

80. Zacharopoulos IP, Papadaki T, Manor RS, Briscoe D. Treatment of idiopathic orbital inflammatory disease with cyclosporine-A: a case presentation. Semin Ophthalmol. 2009;24:260–1.

81. Osborne SF, Sims JL, Rosser PM. Short-term use of Infliximab in a case of recalcitrant idiopathic orbital inflammatory disease. Clin Experiment Ophthalmol. 2009;37:897–900.

82. Smith JR, Rosenbaum JT. A role for methotrexate in the management of non-infectious orbital inflammatory disease. Br J Ophthalmol. 2001;85:1220–4.

83. Hatton MP, Rubin PA, Foster CS. Successful treatment of idiopathic orbital inflammation with mycophenolate mofetil. Am J Ophthalmol. 2005;140(5): 916–8.

84. Eagle K, King A, Fisher C, Souhami R. Cyclophosphamide induced remission in relapsed, progressive idiopathic orbital inflammation ('Pseudotumour'). Clin Oncol (R Coll Radiol). 1995;7: 402–4.

85. Shah SS, Lowder CY, Schmitt MA, Wilke WS, Kosmorsky GS, Meisler DM. Low-dose methotrexate therapy for ocular inflammatory disease. Ophthalmology. 1992;99:1419–23.

IgG₄-Related Orbital Inflammation

3

Victor M. Elner and Hakan Demirci

3.1 Introduction

IgG4-related inflammations are recently recognized fibro-inflammatory conditions, characterized by tumefactive lesions containing dense lymphoplasmacytic infiltrates rich in IgG4+ plasma cells, storiform fibrosis, and obliterative phlebitis that are associated with elevated serum IgG4 [1, 2]. First described by Hamano et al. [3] in 2001, its incidence in Japan is estimated to be 0.28–1.08 cases per 100,000 people [2]. Hamano et al. [3] reported elevated serum IgG4 levels and infiltration of numerous IgG4+ plasma cells in ureteral and pancreatic lesions associated with retroperitoneal fibrosis in patients with autoimmune pancreatitis. In 2003, Kamisawa et al. [4] observed severe or moderate infiltration of IgG4+ plasma cells associated with CD4+ and CD8+ T lymphocytes in autoimmune pancreatitis lesions and in lesions of the liver, stomach, colon, salivary glands, and bone marrow. They proposed a new clinicopathological entity, IgG4-related systemic disease, in which IgG4+ plasma cells extensively infiltrate organs. Since its original observation, IgG4-related inflammation has been reported in almost every tissue with the pancreas, hepatobiliary tract, salivary glands, lymph nodes,

retroperitoneum, and orbit most commonly involved [5, 6]. For each of these tissues, the diagnosis of IgG4-related disease has replaced established clinicopathological diagnoses that were otherwise used for patients meeting the criteria for IgG4-related disease. Meanwhile other patients not meeting the criteria retain the previous clinicopathological diagnoses. Therefore, there are clinicopathological entities with patients divided into those with IgG4-related disease and those that retain the previous established diagnosis for each of the entities. Because this phenomenon affects so many clinicopathological entities, it is likely that the findings used to diagnose IgG4-related disease are really the result of a particular host response rather than a newly recognized disease, a notion that is supported by the strong racial predisposition reported for IgG4-related disease. We therefore prefer to refer the term IgG4-related inflammation to IgG4-related disease.

Orbital and adnexal tissues are the fifth most commonly affected extrapancreatic site and occur in 4–13 % of patients with IgG4-related inflammation [3, 7]. While IgG4-related pancreatitis has a strong male predilection of 2.8–7.5:1, men and women are equally affected with M:F ratio of 1.3:1 in IgG4-related orbital inflammation [5, 7–9]. IgG4-related inflammation has a mean age of onset of 56 years in orbital cases and 58–69 years in pancreatitis cases [8–11]. The frequency of IgG4-related inflammation appears to show racial variations in incidence. For pancreatitis, a review of literature showed that 76 % of cases were from

V.M. Elner, MD, PhD (✉) • H. Demirci, MD
Department of Ophthalmology and Visual Sciences,
W.K. Kellogg Eye Center, University of Michigan,
1000 Wall St, Ann Arbor, MI 48105, USA
e-mail: velner@med.umich.edu;
hdemirci@med.umich.edu

H. Demirci (ed.), *Orbital Inflammatory Diseases and Their Differential Diagnosis*,
Essentials in Ophthalmology, DOI 10.1007/978-3-662-46528-8_3,
© Springer-Verlag Berlin Heidelberg 2015

Japan, South Korea, Hong Kong, and Taiwan and only 16 % of cases were Caucasian [10]. Compared to IgG4-related pancreatitis which is more severe in men, orbital involvement shows that the proportion of cases resistant to one or more treatment modalities is evenly distributed between men and women [8, 9].

Similarly, a review of histopathology slides from 1,014 patients with orbital lymphoproliferative disease in Japan resulted in reclassification of 22 % of cases as IgG4-related disease [12, 13]. The same evaluation was performed in 164 patients with ocular adnexal lymphoproliferative disease in the United States, and only 5 % of them were reclassified as IgG4-related disease [14].

3.2   Clinical Presentation

IgG4-related inflammation can affect any tissue in the orbit including the lacrimal gland, extraocular muscle, sclera, optic nerve, nasolacrimal sac and duct, sensory nerves, eyelid, and rarely conjunctiva [9, 12, 15–21]. A recent review of 65 patients with IgG4-related orbital inflammation showed that lacrimal gland enlargement (88 %) was the most common, followed by trigeminal nerve branch enlargement (39 %), extraocular muscle enlargement (25 %), diffuse infiltration of orbital fat (23 %), orbital mass lesions (17 %), eyelid mass lesions (12 %), and nasolacrimal duct obstructive lesions (2 %) [22]. In up to 52 % of patients, more than one orbital tissue were involved. Patients usually present with a mass or mass-related symptoms including painless eyelid swelling, proptosis with or without diplopia, and mild or no signs of inflammation [9, 15, 16]. A review of literature showed bilateral involvement in 62 % of patients [23]. Visual acuity is usually unaffected, and some patients are asymptomatic with lesions found incidentally on physical examination or imaging studies [9, 15, 16]. On magnetic resonance imaging, orbital lesions are hyperintense on T1-weighted images and hypointense on T2-weighted images. They usually show homogenous enhancement with gadolinium and no destructive bony involvement [17]. Reported is a single case of IgG4-related inflammation with

osteo-destructive lesions that affected the orbital bones and involved the orbital apex, cavernous sinus, palate, nasal septum, turbinates, and paranasal sinuses [15]. A recent study showed that infraorbital nerve involvement associated with enlargement of bony canal strongly suggests IgG4-related inflammation [24].

Orbital cases may be associated with extraorbital inflammatory lesions, most commonly involving salivary glands and lymph nodes [9, 16, 18–20]. FDG-PET is a useful imaging modality for systemic evaluation of IgG4-related inflammation and shows distant and silent sites of involvement [25]. There is a current trend to reclassify the majority of cases of Mikulicz's disease as IgG4-related disease. These individuals demonstrate simultaneous bilateral involvement of the lacrimal glands, submandibular glands, or parotid glands and are considered to be affected by a clinical subtype of IgG4-related disease. Matsui et al. [26] reviewed 25 cases of IgG4-related Mikulicz's disease and found that 44 % of them had asthma and allergic rhinitis, in comparison to allergic rhinitis prevalence of 8–25 % in general Japanese population.

3.3   Diagnosis

Based on two IgG4-related disease study groups organized by the Ministry of Health, Labor and Welfare of Japan, comprehensive clinical diagnostic criteria for IgG4-related disease include (1) clinical examination showing characteristic diffuse/localized swelling or masses in single or multiple organs, (2) hematological evaluation showing elevated serum IgG4 concentrations ($\geq$135 mg/dL), and (3) histopathological examination showing marked lymphocyte and plasma cell infiltration and fibrosis, with IgG4+ plasma cells comprising more than 40 % of the total plasma cell population and with at least 10 IgG4+ plasma cells per high-power microscopic field [2]. However, in some tissues, greater numbers of IgG4+ plasma cells are required for the diagnosis. In lacrimal gland lesions, more than 100 IgG4+ plasma cells/hpf are required [27]. If all three criteria are present, it is classified as definite IgG4-related disease. If the first and third criteria are present, it is probable for IgG4-related disease, and if the first and second criteria are present, it is possible for IgG4-related disease [2]. The presence of IgG4+ plasma cells alone in a biopsy specimen is not specific for IgG4-related disease. Both increased absolute number and proportion of IgG4+ plasma cells are required for the diagnosis. When counting IgG4+ cells, maximum IgG4+ staining areas should be selected and at least three high-power microscopic fields should be averaged [5, 27]. It should be kept in mind that the size of high-power field may change from one microscope to another, but it is generally performed with 40× objective and 10× ocular lenses [9].

Serum IgG4 level varies among the patients who have orbital vs extra-orbital inflammation and unilateral vs bilateral involvement. A review of 27 patients showed that serum IgG4 levels averaged 809 mg/dL in patients with extra-orbital inflammation compared to 235 mg/dL in patients without extra-orbital inflammation and 636 mg/dL in patients with bilateral inflammation compared to 111 mg/dL in patients with unilateral probable disease [15]. The patients with hilar lymphadenopathy or lacrimal and salivary gland lesions were found to have significantly higher IgG4 levels than those without [28]. Elevated serum IgG4 level (>135 mg/dL) is a useful diagnostic tool and has a sensitivity of 97 % and specificity of 79.6 % in diagnosing IgG4-related disease [29]. Serum IgG4 level can be elevated in Churg-Strauss syndrome, multicentric Castleman's disease, eosinophilic disorders, and in some patients with rheumatoid arthritis, systemic sclerosis, chronic hepatitis, and liver cirrhosis [30]. Additionally, 30 % of patients diagnosed with probable IgG4-related disease may have a normal serum IgG4 level [31].

In the setting of proven IgG4-related inflammation elsewhere in the body, ophthalmic inflammatory lesions may present another manifestation of the condition and not require biopsy. Similarly, in the patients with involvement of orbital structures that are difficult to biopsy, such as extraocular muscles, concurrent inflammatory lesions at the non-ocular sites may represent opportunity for biopsy with low morbidity.

3.4 Histopathological Features

The main histopathological features used to diagnose IgG4-related disease are lymphoplasmacytic infiltration, lymphoid follicle formation, obliterative phlebitis, and storiform fibrosis which are accompanied by atrophy and loss of structures within involved tissue [27, 32]. These features vary depending on the tissue and the age of the lesion. The lymphoplasmacytic infiltrate is more intense in early lesions and consists of polyclonal T lymphocytes, IgG4+ plasma cells, and scattered eosinophils. Fibrosis often develops as lesions mature and is accompanied by atrophy. However, some lesions start as a primary sclerosing inflammation [5, 16]. The lack of lymphoplasmacytic infiltrate and predominance of sclerosis or fibrosis often create challenges in histopathological diagnosis because of the paucity of infiltrating leukocytes, including IgG4+ plasma cells. Based on the relative predominance of the lymphoplasmacytic and sclerotic components, IgG4-related disease is subclassified in three categories: pseudolymphomatous, mixed, and sclerotic [33]. In patients with orbital involvement, the mixed pattern is the most common, followed by the sclerotic and pseudolymphomatous which occur with almost equal frequency. Histopathologically, IgG4-related inflammation differs in the orbit and lacrimal gland compared to other tissues with two exceptions. First, the fibrosis within the orbit rarely forms storiform patterns as it does in extra-orbital tissues [27]. Second, obliterative phlebitis is uncommon in the orbit, while it is invariably seen in the pancreatic lesions [1, 11, 12, 32].

3.5 Pathogenesis

The underlying immune mechanisms of IgG4-related inflammation remain unknown. Several studies have been performed to evaluate autoimmunity as a possible cause [34]. Nonspecific antinuclear antibodies have been identified in more than half of patients with IgG4-related inflammation [34]. Antibodies specific for lactoferrin and carbonic anhydrase (CA)-II are the most frequently detected autoantibodies in autoimmune pancreatitis, affecting 73 and 54 % of patients, respectively [35], with a strong correlation between increased serum IgG4 and anti-CA-II antibody levels [35]. Pancreatic secretory trypsin inhibitor is another potential autoantigen which was detected in 30–40 % of patients with IgG4-related autoimmune pancreatitis [34]. Because of the difference in the clinical presentation of IgG4-related pancreatitis and orbital inflammation, it is suggested that the orbital inflammations might be caused by an antigen of the upper respiratory or digestive tracts that affects men and women equally, while the pancreatitis might be caused by an antigen of the lower respiratory or digestive tracts that affects mainly men [9]. Frulloni et al. [36] found that *Helicobacter pylori* surface protein was present in 95 % of patients with autoimmune pancreatitis, suggesting that this antigen might play a role in the pathogenesis of IgG4-related pancreatitis. In a proteomics study, Yamamoto et al. [37] found a 13.1 kDa protein autoantigen in all patients with IgG4-related inflammation, regardless of the organ(s) affected. Taken together, these studies suggest that multiple antigens, including a key autoantigen, may be an initiating factor for IgG4-related inflammation.

Analysis of cytokines expressed in patients with IgG4-related inflammation provided important insights into the pathogenesis of the disorder. Real-time polymerase chain reaction (RT-PCR) shows that significantly increased levels of Th-2 cytokines, namely, IL-4, IL-5, IL-10, and IL-13, as well as a secondary pro-fibrotic cytokines, transforming growth factor (TGF)-beta, and connective tissue growth factor (CTGF) in IgG4-related inflammation of the pancreas [38]. The expression of Foxp3 messenger RNA, a transcription factor specific for naturally arising CD4(+)CD25(+) regulatory T lymphocytes, is also significantly increased in IgG4-related inflammation including orbital inflammatory pseudotumor [20, 38, 39]. A similar study of patients with IgG4-related dacryoadenitis showed that IL-4, IL-5, IL-10, IL-13, and TGF-β, but not Th-1 cytokines, as well as a master upregulator of Th-2 responses, GATA3, were significantly elevated in peripheral blood CD4+ T lymphocytes [40].

Th-2 cells play a role in antibody-mediated immunity, parasitic infections, asthma, and allergy. Treg cells are important in immune tolerance, lymphocyte homeostasis, and downregulation of immune responses. In autoimmune inflammation, Treg cells suppress inflammation via cell-cell contact and secretion of immunosuppressive cytokines, IL-10 and TGF-β, while promoting fibrosis [41, 42]. Th-2 cytokines IL-4, IL-5, IL-6, and IL-13 transform B lymphocytes into plasma cells which produce antibodies, including autoantibodies. These cytokines in conjunction with TGF-beta, CTGF, and IGF-2 stimulate fibroblast proliferation, differentiation, and collagen production necessary for fibrosis. In particular, IL-13 induces TGF-β gene expression via IL-13Rα2 in macrophages, enhancing fibrosis [9]. Th-2 cytokines also stimulate B lymphocytes to produce IL-6 which promotes aforementioned fibroblast activities and is a potent stimulator of plasma cell differentiation and proliferation. Treg cells secrete IL-10 and TGF-beta which promote proliferation and differentiation of B lymphocytes into plasma cells to secrete IgG4 isotype and switching plasma cell secretion from IgE, promoted by Th-2 cytokines, IL-4 and IL-13, to IgG4. Treg cells also regulate other activities of Th-2 cells. Treg secretion of IL-10 and TGF-beta suppresses Th-2 cytokines IL-3, IL-4, and IL-5 which are required for the differentiation, survival, and activity of mast cells, basophils, and eosinophils as well as for homing of Th2 cells. Thus, there is a delicate balance between Th-2 and Treg cells in the evolving inflammatory responses in which eosinophilia, fibrosis, and IgG4 secretion may dominate.

IgG4 constitutes less than 5 % of total IgG and has unique anti-inflammatory properties that may affect all of the various types of immune inflammatory responses [29]. Classically produced in response to parasites and allergens, IgG4 is generated against protein targets but lacks the ability to activate complement and participate in complement mediated lysis and lacks the ability to promote antibody-dependent cell-mediated toxicity or form immune complexes. It also has low affinity for type I (CD64) Fc receptors and no affinity for type II (CD32) or III (CD16) Fc receptors. Furthermore, it has the ability to displace proinflammatory IgG1, IgG3, or IgE antibodies from antigen-binding sites. IgG4 titers increase with the development of antigenic tolerance [1, 43, 44, 45], an effect that is utilized therapeutically as the basis of desensitization of patients to external antigens including peanut, egg, and milk protein antigens who exhibit increase in serum IgG4 level with therapy [46]. These features suggest that IgG4 is a surrogate marker of a particular type of pro-fibrotic inflammatory process in which it serves to mitigate inflammatory responses [9].

In a study of IgG4-related Mikulicz's disease, Yamada et al. [47] demonstrated the effects of Th-2 cytokines in human disease. They found an admixture of polyclonal IgG4+ plasma cells infiltrating lacrimal glands, which they attributed to antigenic responses in which IgE+ and IgG4+ plasma cells undergo Th-2 cytokine-induced class switching thereby retaining overlap of antigen specificity of the generated IgE and IgG4 antibodies. Yamada et al. [47] thought that this was the reason for high incidence of asthma and allergic rhinitis in patients with IgG4-related inflammation. Because they also found genetically related B cells and plasma cells in the lacrimal glands and peripheral blood, Yamada et al. [47] suggested that memory B cells or long-lived plasma cells migrate from lacrimal or salivary glands to the bone marrow or directly to other target organs, causing multiorgan involvement in IgG4-related inflammation.

Therefore, multiple lines of evidence suggest that IgG4-related inflammation may be present in certain susceptible individuals affected by various disease entities of virtually any organ system, while other individuals with the same disease do not demonstrate the features of IgG4-related inflammation. Basis for the tendency toward IgG4-related inflammation is a particular Th-2-mediated inflammatory response that may be initiated by particular autoantigens that become recognized during the inflammatory process. The pathogenesis of IgG4-related inflammation also clarifies the molecular basis

of clinical and histopathological findings that have been reported to characterize the disease, namely, inflammatory masses, elevated serum IgG4, lymphoplasmacytic infiltration, lymphoid follicle formation, predominance of IgG4+ plasma cells, and fibrosis. It is not surprising that these findings vary from patient to patient depending on organ systems involved and stage of the diseases in which they are present.

3.6 Differential Diagnosis

The differential diagnosis of IgG4-related disease has been reported to include most other orbital inflammatory conditions, including idiopathic orbital inflammation, Wegener's granulomatosis, sarcoidosis, Sjögren syndrome, and systemic lupus erythematosus, in which some of the criteria for IgG4-related disease have been reported. There are several reports of IgG4-related inflammation in patients with idiopathic inflammatory pseudotumor, indicating that a minority of these patients fulfill the criteria that required for IgG4-related disease [19]. For Wegener's granulomatosis, >30 IgG4+ plasma cells per high-power field and >40 % IgG4+/IgG+ were reported in 31 % of patients [48]. Sarcoidosis which can have similar clinical findings of orbital, lung, and lymph node involvement was reported to have elevated serum IgG4 levels in 8 % of patients [49]. Similarly, about 8 % of patients with Sjögren syndrome were found to have increased IgG4 serum levels accompanied by bilateral salivary and lacrimal gland involvement [50]. About 14 % of patients with systemic lupus erythematosus have increased IgG4 serum levels.

Review of the literature suggests that patients with IgG4-related orbital inflammation have a higher risk of developing orbital lymphoma [9, 12, 14, 20, 51]. In two series of IgG4-related orbital disease, 14 and 11 % of patients developed orbital lymphoma [12, 20]. This is higher than that observed in other organs affected by IgG4-related disease [52]. In the literature, 21 cases of ocular adnexal lymphoma have been reported to have abundant IgG4+ plasma cells and IgG4/IgG ratios >40 % [9, 12, 14, 20, 51]. In IgG4-related orbital inflammation, the most commonly associated ocular adnexal lymphoma is extranodal marginal zone B-cell lymphoma. The histopathological differences between IgG4-related MALT lymphoma of the ocular adnexa and other lymphomas include the rarity of lymphoepithelial lesions, the presence of fibrosis, and the coexistence of IgG4+ plasma cells in IgG4-related MALT lymphomas [9, 12, 51]. The mechanism of lymphomagenesis in IgG4-related inflammation is suggested to be related to chronic antigenic stimulation-driven lymphoid proliferation [9, 12, 51, 53], the lymphoma originating from preserved lymphoid follicles within the tissue undergoing progressive fibrosis.

3.7   Treatment

Treatment options include corticosteroids and other immunosuppressive drugs, radiotherapy, and rituximab [9, 15]. Outcomes of different treatment approaches are usually based on retrospective, observational studies, rather than prospective, randomized clinical trials [9]. Sato et al [12] observed three patients with IgG4-related orbital disease without systemic involvement and found that the disease remained stable in two patients and spontaneously regressed in the other after a mean follow-up of 38 months. IgG4-related disease almost always shows a good initial response to corticosteroids, especially in the early phase of the disease; in fact, the diagnosis of IgG4-related disease is suspect in those who do not initially respond to corticosteroids. However, the effectiveness of corticosteroids is often transient. As the disease evolves into more sclerotic phase, disease becomes more recalcitrant to corticosteroid therapy. The dose and length of corticosteroid treatment may vary depend on the patient's response and treatment protocol. The consensus protocol for IgG4-related pancreatitis is an initial induction oral dosage of 0.6 mg/kg/day for 2–4 weeks, followed by tapering 5 mg/day every 1–2 weeks based on clinical manifestations, blood tests (liver enzymes and IgG4 levels), and imaging [54]. A review of the literature showed that

half of the cases of IgG4-related orbital disease who are initially treated with corticosteroids had recurrence of symptoms during the follow-up period [9], leading to the conclusion that there is insufficient data to detect a correlation between the degree of fibrosis and corticosteroid resistance in IgG4-related orbital disease. A recent study showed that patients with orbital disease and positive serologic tests for rheumatoid factor showed a significantly higher risk of relapse after corticosteroid therapy [55]. In IgG4-related pancreatitis, a remission maintenance therapy of 2.5–5 mg/day is recommended for over 2–3 months. This is shown to decrease the recurrence rate of IgG4-related pancreatitis from 92 to 23 % at 3 years [56, 57]. Immunosuppressants have been used in the cases that are resistant to oral corticosteroid therapy. A review of the literature reported that corticosteroid-sparing immunosuppressive therapy used in seven cases of orbital disease resulted in complete response in only two patients [9]. Thus, azathioprine, methotrexate, and mycophenolate mofetil have limited success in the treatment of IgG4-related disease [58]. Khosroshahi et al. [59] reviewed their experiences with rituximab therapy (2 infusions of 1,000 mg, 15 days apart) in ten patients who were refractory to corticosteroids and immunosuppressive therapy. Nine of ten patients showed clinical improvement and significant decrease in IgG4 levels within 1 month of rituximab therapy, and all ten patients were able to discontinue corticosteroid and other immunosuppressive therapy. Two of the patients had flares associated with normalization of circulating B cells and concomitant elevations of IgG4 serum levels; both responded to repeat courses of rituximab infusion. A review of the literature showed that 8 cases treated with external beam radiotherapy had variable results [12]. Of 8 cases, 5 cases showed complete response, 2 cases had partial response, and 1 case relapsed after external beam radiotherapy.

Compliance with Ethical Requirements Victor M. Elner and Hakan Demirci declare that they have no conflict of interest.

No human or animal studies were carried out for this article.

References

1. Stone JH, Zen V, Deshpande V. IgG4-related disease. N Engl J Med. 2012;386:539–51.
2. Umehara H, Okazaki K, Masaki Y, et al. Comprehensive diagnostic criteria for IgG4-related disease. Mod Rheumatol. 2011;22:21–30.
3. Hamano H, Kawa S, Horiuchi A, Unno H, Furuya N, Akamatsu T, et al. High serum IgG4 concentrations in patients with sclerosing pancreatitis. N Engl J Med. 2001;344:732–8.
4. Kamisawa T, Funata N, Hayashi Y, Eishi Y, Koike M, Tsuruta K, et al. A new clinicopathological entity of IgG4-related autoimmune disease. J Gastroenterol. 2003;38:982–4.
5. Divatia M, Kim SA, Ro Y. IgG4-related sclerosing disease, an emerging entity: a review of a multi-system disease. Yonsei Med J. 2012;53:15–34.
6. Carruthers MN, Stone JH, Khosroshahi A. The latest on IgG4-related disease: a rapidly emerging disease. Curr Opin Rheumatol. 2012;24:60–9.
7. Takuma K, Kamisawa T, Anjiki H, Egawa N, Igarashi Y. Metachronous extrapancreatic lesions in autoimmune pancreatitis. Intern Med. 2010;49:529–33.
8. Nishimori I, Tamakoshi A, Otsuki M. Prevalence of autoimmune pancreatitis in Japan from a nationwide survey in 2002. J Gastroenterol. 2007;42:6–8.
9. Andrew N, Kearney D, Selva D. IgG4-related orbital disease: a meta-analysis and review. Acta Ophalmol. 2013;91:694–700.
10. Masaki Y, Dong L, Kurose N, et al. Proposal for a new clinical entity, IgG4-positive multiorgan lympho-proliferative syndrome: analysis of 64 cases of IgG4-related disorders. Ann Rheum Dis. 2009;68:1310–5.
11. Khosrashahi A, Stone JH. A clinical overview of IgG4-related systemic disease. Curr Opin Rheumatol. 2011;23:57–66.
12. Sato Y, Ohshima K, Ichimura K, et al. Ocular adnexal IgG4-related disease has uniform clinicopathology. Pathol Int. 2008;58:465–70.
13. Japanese study group of IgG4-related ophthalmic disease. A prevalence study of IgG4-related ophthalmic disease in Japan. Jpn J Ophthalmol. 2013;57:573–9.
14. Karamchandani JR, Younes SF, Warnke RA, Natkunam Y. IgG4-related systemic sclerosing disease of the ocular adnexa: a potential mimic of ocular lymphoma. Am J Clin Pathol. 2012;137:699–711.
15. Wallace ZS, Deshpande V, Stone JH. Ophthalmic manifestations of IgG4-related disease: single-center experience and literature review. Semin Arthritis Rheum. 2014;43:806–17.
16. Cheuk W, Yuen HK, Chan JK. Chronic sclerosing dacryoadenitis: part of the spectrum of IgG4-related sclerosing disease? Am J Surg Pathol. 2007;31:643–5.
17. Toyoda K, Oba H, Kutomi K, et al. MR imaging of IgG4-related disease in the head and neck and brain. AJNR Am J Neuroradiol. 2012;33:2136–9.
18. Matsuo T, Ichimura K, Sato Y, Tanimoto Y, Kiura K, Kanazawa S, Okada T, Yoshino T. Immunoglobulin G4 (IgG4-)-positive or –negative ocular adnexal benign lymphoid lesions in relation to systemic involvement. J Clin Exp Hematop. 2010;50:129–42.
19. Plaza JA, Garrity JA, Dogan A, Ananthamurthy A, Witzig TE, Salomao DR. Orbital inflammation with IgG4-positive plasma cells: manifestation of IgG4 systemic disease. Arch Ophthalmol. 2011;129: 421–8.
20. Go H, Kim JE, Kim YA, Chung HK, Khwarg SI, Kim CW, Jeon YK. Ocular adnexal IgG4-related disease: comparative analysis with mucosa-associated lymphoid tissue lymphoma and other chronic inflammatory conditions. Histopathology. 2012;60:296–312.
21. Paulus YM, Cockerham KP, Cockerham GC, Gratzinger D. IgG4-positive sclerosing orbital inflammation involving the conjunctiva: a case report. Ocul Immunol Inflamm. 2012;20:375–7.
22. Sogabe Y, Ohshima K, Azumi A, Takahira M, Kase S, Tsuji H, Yashikawa H, Nakamura T. Location and frequency of lesions in patients with IgG4-related ophthalmic disease. Graefes Arch Clin Exp Ophthalmol. 2014;252:531–8.
23. Mulay K, Aggarwal E, Jariwala M, Honavar S. Orbital immunoglobulin –G4-related disease: case series and literature review. Clin Experiment Ophthalmol. 2014;42:682–7. Doi 10.111.
24. Hardy TG, McNabb AA, Rose GE. Enlargement of the infraorbital nerve: an important sign associated with orbital reactive lymphoid hyperplasia or immunoglobulin G4-related disease. Ophthalmology. 2014;121:1297–303.
25. Himi T, Takano K, Yamamoto M, et al. A novel concept of Mikulicz's disease as IgG4-related disease. Auris Nasus Larynx. 2012;39:9–17.
26. Matsui S, Taki H, Shinoda K, et al. Respiratory involvement in IgG4-related Mikulicz's disease. Mod Rheumatol. 2012;22:31–9.
27. Deshpande V, Zen Y, Chan JK, et al. Consensus statement on the pathology of IgG4-related disease. Mod Pathol. 2012;25:1181–92.
28. Hamano H, Arakura N, Muraki T, Ozaki Y, Kiyosawa K, Kawa S. Prevalence and distribution of extrapancreatic lesions complicating autoimmune pancreatitis. J Gastroenterol. 2006;41:1197–205.
29. Masaki Y, Kurose N, Yamamoto M, Takahashi H, Saeki T, Azumi A, et al. Cutoff values of serum IgG4 and histopathological IgG4+ plasma cells for diagnosis of patients with IgG4-related disease. Int J Rheumatol. 2012;2012:580814.
30. Yamamoto M, Tabeya T, Naishiro Y, Yajima H, Ishigami K, Shimizu Y, et al. Value of serum IgG4 in the diagnosis of IgG4-related disease and in differentiation from rheumatic disease and other diseases. Mod Rheumatol. 2012;22:419.
31. Ebbo M, Daniel L, Pavic M, Seve P, Hamidou M, Andres E, et al. IgG4-related systemic disease: features and treatment response in a French cohort: results of a multicenter registry. Medicine (Baltimore). 2012;91:49–56.

32. Smyrk TC. Pathological features of IgG4-related sclerosing disease. Curr Opin Rheumatol. 2011;23:74–9.

33. Cheuk W, Chan J. IgG4-related sclerosing disease: a critical appraisal of an evolving clinicopathologic entity. Adv Anat Pathol. 2010;17:303–32.

34. Zen Y, Nakanuma Y. Pathogenesis of IgG4-related disease. Curr Opin Rheumatol. 2011;23:114–8.

35. Okazaki K, Uchida K, Ohana M, et al. Autoimmune pancreatitis is associated with autoantibodies and a Th1/Th2-type cellular immune response. Gastroenterology. 2000;118:573–81.

36. Frulloni L, Lunardi C, Simone R, et al. Identification of a novel antibody associated with autoimmune pancreatitis. N Engl J Med. 2009;381:2135–42.

37. Yamamoto M, Naishiro Y, Suzuki C, et al. Proteomics analysis in 28 patients with systemic IgG4-related plasmacytic syndrome. Rheumatol Int. 2010;30:565–8.

38. Zen Y, Fujii T, Harada K, et al. Th2 and regulatory immune reactions are increased in immunoglobulin G4-related sclerosing pancreatitis and cholangitis. Hepatology. 2007;45:1538–46.

39. Koyabu M, Uchida K, Miyoshi H, et al. Analysis of regulatory T cells and IgG4-positive plasma cells among patient of IgG4-related sclerosing cholangitis and autoimmune live diseases. J Gastroenterol. 2010;45:732–41.

40. Kanari H, Kagami S, Kashiwakuma D, et al. Role of Th2 cells in IgG4-related lacrimal gland enlargement. Int Arch Allergy Immunol. 2010;152:47–53.

41. Cools N, Ponsaerts P, van Tendeloo VF, et al. Regulatory T cells and human disease. Clin Dev Immunol. 2007;2007:89195.

42. Sakaguchi S. Naturally arising CD4+ regulatory T cells for immunologic self-tolerance and negative control of immune responses. Annu Rev Immunol. 2004;22:531–62.

43. Lock RJ, Unsworth DJ. Immunoglobulins and immunoglobulin subclasses in the elderly. Ann Clin Biochem. 2003;40:143–8.

44. Nirula A, Glaser SM, Kalled SL, Taylor FR. What is IgG4? A review of the biology of a unique immunoglobulin subtype. Curr Opin Rheumatol. 2011;23:119–24.

45. Lighaam LC, Aalberse RC, Rispens T. IgG4-related fibrotic diseases from an immunological perspective: regulators out of control? Int J Rheumatol. 2012;2012:789164.

46. Mousallem T, Burks AW. Immunology in the clinic review series; focus on allergies: immunotherapy for food allergy. Clin Exp Immunol. 2012;167:26–31.

47. Yamada K, Kawano M, Inoue R, et al. Clonal relationship between infiltrating immunoglobulin G4 (IgG4)-positive plasma cells in lacrimal glands and circulating IgG4-positive lymphocytes in Mikulicz's disease. Clin Exp Immunol. 2008;152:432–9.

48. Chang SY, Keogh K, Lewis J, Ryu J, Yi E. Increased IgG4-positive plasma cells in granulomatosis with polyangiitis: a diagnostic pitfall of IgG4-related disease. Int J Rheumatol. 2012;2012:121702.

49. Tsushima K, Yokoyama T, Kawa S, Hamano H, Tanabe T, Koizumi T, Honda T, Kawakami S, Kubo K. Elevated IgG4 levels in patients demonstrating sarcoidosis-like radiologic findings. Medicine (Baltimore). 2011;90:194–200.

50. Mavragani CP, Fragoulis GE, Rontogianni D, Kanariou M, Moutsopoulos HM. Elevated IgG4 serum levels among primary sjogren's syndrome patients: do they unmask underlying IgG4-related disease? Arthritis Care Res. 2014;66:773–7.

51. Cheuk W, Yuen HK, Chan AC, et al. Ocular adnexal lymphoma associated with IgG4+ chronic sclerosing dacryoadenitis: a previously undescribed complication of IgG4-related sclerosing disease. Am J Surg Pathol. 2008;32:1159–67.

52. Takahashi N, Ghazale AH, Smyrk TC, Mandrekar JN, Chari ST. Possible association between IgG4-associated systemic disease with or without autoimmune pancreatitis and non-Hodgkin lymphoma. Pancreas. 2009;38:523–6.

53. Kanda G, Ryu T, Shirai T, Ijichi M, Hishima T, Kitamura S, Bandai Y. Peripheral T-cell lymphoma that developed during the follow-up of IgG4-related disease. Intern Med. 2011;50:155–60.

54. Kamisawa T, Okazaki K, Kawa S, et al. Amendment of the Japanese consensus guidelines for autoimmune pancreatitis, 2013 III. Treatment and prognosis of autoimmune pancreatitis. J Gastroenterol. 2014;49:961–70.

55. Kubota T, Katayama M, Moritani S, Yoshino T. Serologic factors in early relapse of IgG4-related orbital inflammation after steroid treatment. Am J Ophthalmol. 2013;155:373–6.

56. Kim HM, Chung MJ, Chunk JB. Remission and relapse of autoimmune pancreatitis: focusing on corticosteroid treatment. Pancreas. 2010;39:555–60.

57. Kamisawa T, Shimosegawa T, Okazaki K, et al. Standard steroid treatment for autoimmune pancreatitis. Gut. 2009;58:1504–7.

58. Khosroshahi A, Stone JH. Treatment approaches to IgG4-related systemic disease. Curr Opin Rheumatol. 2011;23:67–71.

59. Khosroshahi A, Carruthers MN, Deshpande V, Unizony S, Bloch DB, Stone JH. Rituximab for the treatment of IgG4-related disease: lessons from 10 consecutive patients. Medicine. 2012;91:57–66.

Orbital and Adnexal Sarcoidosis

4

Hakan Demirci

4.1 Introduction

Sarcoidosis is an idiopathic, autoimmune granulomatous disorder that is characterized by noncaseating granulomata on histopathologic examination [1]. Although it can affect any race, gender, and age, most studies report a peak incidence in adults between the ages of 20 and 39 years for both genders and second peak incidence at age 65–69 in women [2]. Age-adjusted annual incidence rate is estimated to be 3–10 per 100,000 for Caucasians and 35–80 per 100,000 for African-Americans in the USA, 15–20 per 100,000 in the Northern Europe, 1–5 per 100,000 in Southern Europe, and 1–2 per 100,000 in Japan [2]. Although sarcoidosis can affect any organ, intrathoracic presentation such as hilar and mediastinal lymphadenopathy or lung involvement is seen in more than 90 % of patients. Skin and eye involvements are the next common extrathoracic presentations in 20–30 % and 20–25 % of patients, respectively [3]. In the ACCESS (A Case Control Etiologic Study of Sarcoidosis) study in which 706 newly diagnosed patients and an equal number of age-, race-, and sex-matched control subjects are recruited in ten centers, ocular involvement was more frequent in African-American patients than in Caucasians, and eye involvement was more common in females than males at 13.9 and 8.2 %, respectively [4]. Organ involvement is typically defined at presentation. In the ACCESS study, only 23 % of patients developed one or more new organ involvement during a 2-year follow-up evaluation [5].

4.2 Pathogenesis

In recent years, the pathogenesis of sarcoidosis has been better understood. Sarcoid granulomas are composed of epithelioid cells, mononuclear cells, and CD4 T cells with a few CD8 T cells around the periphery. Bronchoalveolar lavage of sarcoidosis patients showed CD4/CD8 T-cell ratio more than 3–5:1 compared with a ratio of 2:1 in healthy people [6]. Similarly, CD4/CD8 ratios of vitreal and peripheral T lymphocytes were significantly higher in patients with ocular sarcoidosis than in patients without sarcoidosis [7]. In sarcoidosis, the granulomatous inflammation is associated with upregulation of cytokines such as interferon (IFN)-γ, interleukin (IL)-12, IL-18, and IL-27 produced by TH1 cells, consistent with TH1 cell polarization [8–11]. On the other hand, cytokines such as IL-4 and IL-5 produced by TH2 cells are downregulated [9–12].

Environmental factors are associated with increased risk of sarcoidosis. In the ACCESS study, occupational exposure to insecticides,

H. Demirci, MD
Department of Ophthalmology and Visual Science,
W.K. Kellogg Eye Center, University of Michigan,
Ann Arbor, MI, USA
e-mail: hdemirci@umich.edu

H. Demirci (ed.), *Orbital Inflammatory Diseases and Their Differential Diagnosis*,
Essentials in Ophthalmology, DOI 10.1007/978-3-662-46528-8_4,
© Springer-Verlag Berlin Heidelberg 2015

pesticides, or mold and/or mildew and agricultural employment were associated with a 1.5-fold increase in sarcoidosis risk [13]. On the other hand, tobacco use was associated with decreased risk. The authors concluded that there was no single cause of sarcoidosis; rather, the disease is triggered by multiple factors. Genetic and host factors are important in the pathogenesis. Among siblings, all first-degree and second-degree relatives of sarcoidosis patients, the risk of developing sarcoidosis increased fivefold [13]. The genetic basis of sarcoidosis involves the class 2 human leukocyte antigens (HLAs) genes within the MHC locus on chromosome 6 [13, 14]. HLAs are cell surface proteins that are essential for immune recognition and function. In the ACCESS study, the *HLA-DRB1*1101, RB1*0402, DRB1*1201, DRB1*1501, DRB3*0101, DPB1-V76*, and *DRB1*1401* were identified as risk factors for sarcoidosis [15, 16]. Among these HLA alleles, *HLA-DRB1*0401* was associated with increased risk for ocular involvement. Genome-wide association studies identified polymorphisms in the *BTNL2* gene within the MHC locus that are associated with increased risk of sarcoidosis. It is thought that these polymorphisms may influence T-lymphocyte activation and regulation [14].

The clinical and histopathological similarities to tuberculosis have raised questions about the role of mycobacterial organisms in the pathogenesis of sarcoidosis. Although histopathologic studies failed to reveal any microbial organisms, PCR studies showed a 10-fold to 20-fold greater likelihood of detecting mycobacterial DNA in tissues from patients with sarcoidosis than normal controls [17]. Mass spectrometry and protein immunoblotting experiments identified the mycobacterial catalase-peroxidase (mKatG) protein in almost half of patients with sarcoidosis [18]. The mKatG is a virulence factor for *Mycobacterium tuberculosis* and an enzyme that converts the prodrug isoniazid, an antituberculosis agent, to its active microbicidal form. The mKatG is an immunodominant T-cell antigen that causes increased lung and blood CD4 and CD8 T-cell responses in sarcoidosis patients [18–20].

Serum amyloid A (SAA), an amyloid precursor and acute-phase reactant, is both a component and innate regulator of granulomatous inflammation in sarcoidosis through Toll-like receptor-2 [21]. It is expressed at higher levels in sarcoidosis granulomas than in other granulomatous disorders [21]. Additionally, SAA induced granulomatous lung inflammation in animal models and stimulated the expression of cytokines such as IFN-γ, tumor necrosis factor (TNF), and IL-10 [21]. Based on these findings, Chen and Moller [22] proposed that the pathobiology of sarcoidosis is determined by aberrant innate response that results in the induction, misfolding, and aggregation of SAA. According to their hypothetical model [21, 22], in genetically susceptible patients, both etiologic triggers and environmental factors induce innate immune response that leads to expression of systemic and intracellular misfolded and/or aggregated SAA and hyperpolarized TH1 response. The misfolded and/or aggregation of SAA provides a nidus and template for further SAA aggregation in sarcoidosis granuloma. Additionally, SAA and SAA peptides released from granulomas stimulate macrophages and T cells, which results in further secretion of cytokines such as IFN-γ, TNF, IL-12, IL-18, and IL-27 by TH1 cells. Clearance of aggregated SAA and local pathogenic antigen and downregulation of TH1 cell response lead to remission, while inability to clear SAA and local pathogenic antigens leads to chronic inflammation and fibrosis.

4.3   Clinical Features

The percentage of sarcoidosis patients with eye involvement varies widely, depending on racial origin, geographical location, and the diagnostic criteria used for ocular involvement. In a comparative analysis of 571 Finnish and 686 Japanese patients, Pientinalho et al. [23] reported that at presentation, 5 % of Finish patients had eye symptoms, while 41 % of Japanese patients had eye symptoms. In the ACCESS study, African-Americans and females experienced a higher percentage of ocular involvement [13].

Sarcoidosis can involve any part of the eye, including the eyelid, orbit, lacrimal gland, conjunctiva, intraocular structures, and optic nerve. The most common ocular finding is granulomatous uveitis, affecting 20–70 % of patients [24]. Smith and Foster [25] reviewed their experience with 43 ocular sarcoidosis patients and found that anterior uveitis was the most common ocular finding (73 %), followed by vitritis (62 %), retinal and choroidal lesions (34 %), and ocular adnexal and orbital lesions (10 %). In a review of 379 patients with systemic sarcoidosis, Demirci and Christianson [26] reported that 8 % had orbital and adnexal involvement. Orbital manifestations of sarcoidosis are palpable periocular mass (89 %), proptosis (42 %), discomfort (31 %), ptosis (27 %), restricted ocular motility (23 %), dry eye (19 %), diplopia (15 %), and decreased vision (12 %) [27]. Patients with orbital sarcoidosis usually don't develop intraocular inflammation. In a review of 20 patients with orbital sarcoid, Marvrikakis and Rootman [28] reported that anterior uveitis was present in 10 % of the patients. In the literature, the intraocular involvement ranged from 0 to 23 % of the patients with orbital sarcoidosis [26, 27]. In the orbit and adnexa, sarcoidosis most commonly affects the lacrimal gland (42 %), followed by the orbital tissue (39 %), eyelid (12 %), and lacrimal sac (8 %) [27]. In some studies, up to 60 % of patients develop lacrimal gland involvement [29]. The lacrimal gland involvement can present as enlargement of the gland or dry eyes. When sarcoidosis affects the extralacrimal orbital tissue, it presents as diffuse involvement or discrete mass. The discrete mass mostly affects the inferior quadrant [27]. Rarely, sarcoidosis can affect extraocular muscles, which could be symptomatic or asymptomatic [28]. When symptomatic, sarcoidosis presents with painful, external ophthalmoplegia, painless diplopia, or ptosis [28, 30–33]. The other rare orbital presentation is the dural involvement of the optic nerve sheath [28, 34]. Orbital and adnexal sarcoidosis can be the initial sign of the systemic disease, develop in patients with known systemic disease, or affect only orbital and adnexal tissue without developing systemic disease. The term "sarcoidal reaction" or "orbital sarcoid" is used for patients with orbital involvement alone and no systemic sarcoidosis [28]. In a review of 18 patents with orbital sarcoid, Mavrikakis and Rootman [28] reported that systemic sarcoidosis was discovered in half of the patients, while the other half showed no evidence of systemic disease during the mean follow-up of 5 years. In a review of 30 patients with orbital and adnexal sarcoidosis, Demirci and Christianson [26] found that 37 % of patients had known systemic disease, orbital and adnexal involvement was the initial manifestation of systemic disease in 34 % of the patients, and 29 % of patients had disease limited to the region. Using Kaplan-Meier estimates, systemic sarcoidosis was expected in 8 % of the patients who presented with only orbital and adnexal disease by 5 years [26]. No clinical feature was found to be significantly predictive of systemic disease in univariate or multivariate analyses [26].

4.4   Diagnostic Evaluation

Imaging of orbital sarcoidosis demonstrates homogenous or lobular enlargement of the lacrimal gland which molds to the eye or diffuse homogeneous involvement of orbital soft tissue. The involved tissue shows enhancement with contrast in computed tomography or gadolinium in magnetic resonance imaging. On histopathological examination, noncaseating granulomatous inflammation is the hallmark pathologic feature. The granulomata are predominantly composed of epithelioid histiocytes with scattered giant cells and foci of necrosis. Granulomata are usually surrounded by a paucity of lymphoid cells and fibrosis, the so-called naked granulomata.

The diagnosis of orbital sarcoidosis is usually based on clinical and radiologic findings; however, biopsy is required to confirm the diagnosis histopathologically and to exclude other possible diseases. However, even in cases with typical histopathologic findings, other causes of granulomatous inflammation should be ruled out. An international workshop in 2006 provided consensus and established criteria for the clinical diagnosis of ocular sarcoidosis [8]. However, there are no established criteria for clinical diagnosis of orbital sarcoidosis. A complete medical evaluation should be part of the work-up; the orbital specialist should have a high level of suspicion and low threshold for referral to an internist or pulmonologist in the context of findings suspicious for the disease. Skin lesions including erythema nodosum, lupus pernio, lesions along scars, tattoos and prior trauma sites, parotid enlargement, lymphadenopathy, hepatosplenomegaly, neurological signs especially for cranial nerve VII palsy, and normal lung examination are usual clinical findings in suspected cases [35]. Basic laboratory tests ordered in suspected sarcoidosis cases include chest-ray, complete blood count, renal function, serum calcium, liver function tests, tuberculin skin test, 24-h urine test for calcium levels, pulmonary function test, total immunoglobulins, and electrocardiogram. Elevated serum angiotensin-converting enzyme (ACE) level is associated with active sarcoidosis and has 60–73 % sensitivity in diagnosing sarcoidosis [36–38]. However, some recent studies showed no association between elevated ACE levels on ocular presentation [39]. Conjunctival biopsy has been reported to be helpful for the diagnosis of systemic sarcoidosis [40–42], but biopsy of clinically or radiologically involved tissue has a much higher diagnostic yield for sarcoidosis or diseases in the differential diagnosis.

4.5   Management

Management of orbital sarcoidosis usually depends on the symptoms and clinical findings of the patient and involved organs. Spontaneous resolution is observed in up to 60 % of patients with systemic sarcoidosis; however, there is no data regarding the natural history of orbital sarcoidosis [43]. Immunosuppression is the mainstay of treatment for orbital sarcoidosis. Corticosteroids have been the traditional standard of care for severe systemic sarcoidosis, and corticosteroid-sparing agents, such as azathioprine and methotrexate, or antimalarials (chloroquine or hydroxychloroquine) have been used successfully in many cases. In orbital cases without active systemic disease, a course of oral prednisone starting at 1 mg per kilogram of

body weight and tapered over 3 months may be considered as initial therapy. In those who fail to respond or are corticosteroid intolerant, cytotoxic corticosteroid-sparing agents may be used. Despite the widespread use of corticosteroids, there is little evidence of long-term benefits. Resolution of symptoms was reported in 10–20 % of patients who used systemic corticosteroid therapy [43]. In localized orbital disease, periocular corticosteroids (1-ml injection of triamcinolone acetonide 40 mg/mL) may be considered. In a multicentric study of 26 patients with orbital and adnexal sarcoidosis, Prabhakaran et al. [27] reported that 73 % of patients were treated with systemic corticosteroids and 15 % required additional systemic methotrexate therapy. Overall, 85 % of these patients showed a good response to therapy. Demirci and Christianson [26] observed that 93 % of orbital and adnexal sarcoidosis patients regressed or remained stable following systemic corticosteroid therapy after a mean follow-up of 44 months. The long-term effects of immunosuppression on the natural history of the disease are unclear. In a review of seven ocular sarcoidosis patients who had persistent inflammation despite systemic immunosuppressive therapy, Baughman et al. [44] reported significant improvement in all seven patients with antitumor necrosis factor alpha agent infliximab. On the other hand, the antitumor necrosis factor alpha agent etanercept failed to control ocular sarcoidosis [45]. Either infliximab or etanercept has not been used in the management of orbital sarcoidosis.

Compliance with Ethical Requirements Hakan Demirci declares that he has no conflict of interest.

No human or animal studies were carried out by the authors for this article.

References

1. Statement on sarcoidosis. Joint Statement of the American Thoracic Society (ATS), the European Respiratory Society (ERS), and the World Association of Sarcoidosis and Other Granulomatous Disorders (WASOG) adopted by the ATS Board of Directors and by the ERS Executive Committee, February 1999. Am J Respir Crit Care Med. 1999;160:736–55.

2. Rybicki BA, Iannuzzi MC. Epidemiology of sarcoidosis: recent advances and future prospects. Semin Respir Crit Care Med. 2007;28:22–35.
3. Chen ES, Moller DR. Sarcoidosis – scientific progress and clinical challenges. Nat Rev Rheumatol. 2011;7: 457–67.
4. Baughman RP, Teirstein AS, Judson MA, et al. Clinical characteristics of patients in a case control study of sarcoidosis. Am J Respir Crit Care Med. 2001;164:1885–9.
5. Judson MA, Baughman RP, Thompson BW, et al. Two year prognosis of sarcoidosis: the ACCESS experience. Sarcoidosis Vasc Diffuse Lung Dis. 2003; 20:204–11.
6. Walker L, Jorres RA, Costabel U, Magnussen H. Predictive value of BAL cell differentials in the diagnosis of interstitial lung diseases. Eur Respir J. 2004;24:1000–6.
7. Kojima K, Maruyama K, Inaba T, et al. The CD4/CD8 ratio in vitreous fluid is of high diagnostic value in sarcoidosis. Ophthalmology. 2012;119:2386–92.
8. Zissel G, Prasse A, Muller-Quernheim J. Sarcoidosis-immunopathogenetic concepts. Semin Respir Crit Care Med. 2007;28:3–14.
9. Moller DR, Forman JD, Liu MC, et al. Enhanced expression of IL-12 associated with TH1 cytokine profiles in active pulmonary sarcoidosis. J Immunol. 1996;156:4952–60.
10. Greene CM, Meachery G, Taggart CC, et al. Role of IL-18 in CD4 T lymphocyte activation in sarcoidosis. J Immunol. 2000;165:4718–24.
11. Larousserie F, Pflanz S, Coulomb-L'Hermine A, et al. Expression of IL-27 in human TH1-associated granulomatous diseases. J Pathol. 2004;202:164–71.
12. Walker C, Bauer W, Braun RK, et al. Activated T cells and cytokines in bronchoalveolar lavages from patients with various lung diseases associated with eosinophilia. Am J Respir Crit Care Med. 1994; 150:1038–48.
13. Newman LS, Rose CS, Bresnitz EA, et al. A case control etiologic study of sarcoidosis: environmental and occupational risk factors. Am J Respir Crit Care Med. 2004;170:1324–30.
14. Schurmann M, Lympany PA, Reichel P, et al. Familial sarcoidosis is linked to the major histocompatibility complex region. Am J Respir Crit Care Med. 2000; 162:862–4.
15. Morgenthau AS, Iannuzzi MC. Recent advances in sarcoidosis. Chest. 2011;139:174–82.
16. Rossman MD, Thompson B, Frederick M, et al. HLA-DRB1*1101: a significant risk factor for sarcoidosis in blacks and whites. Am J Hum Genet. 2003;73: 720–35.
17. Gupta D, Agarwal R, Agarwal AN, Jindal SK. Molecular evidence for the role of mycobacteria in sarcoidosis: a meta-analysis. Eur Respir J. 2007;30:508–16.
18. Song Z, Marzilli L, Greenlee BM, et al. Mycobacterial catalase-peroxidase is a tissue antigen and target of the adaptive immune response in systemic sarcoidosis. J Exp Med. 2005;201:755–67.
19. Chen ES, Wahlstrom J, Song Z, et al. T cell responses to mycobacterial catalase-peroxidase profile a pathogenic antigen in systemic sarcoidosis. J Immunol. 2008;181:8784–96.
20. Drake WP, Dhason MS, Nadaf M, et al. Cellular recognition of mycobacterium tuberculosis ESAT-6 and KatG peptides in systemic sarcoidosis. Infect Immun. 2007;75:527–30.
21. Chen ES, Song Z, Willett MH, et al. Serum amyloid A regulates granulomatous inflammation in sarcoidosis through Toll-like receptor-2. Am J Respir Crit Care Med. 2010;181:360–3.
22. Chen ES, Moller DR. Etiology of sarcoidosis. Clin Chest Med. 2008;29:365–77.
23. Pietinalho A, Ohmichi M, Hiraga Y, Lofroos AB, Selroos O. The mode of presentation of sarcoidosis in Finland and Hokkaido, Japan. A comparative analysis of 571 Finnish and 686 Japanese patients. Sarcoidosis Vasc Diffuse Lung Dis. 1996;13:159–66.
24. Baughman RP, Lower EE, Kaufman AH. Ocular sarcoidosis. Semin Respir Crit Care Med. 2010;31: 452–62.
25. Smith JA, Foster CS. Sarcoidosis and its ocular manifestations. Int Ophthalmol Clin. 1996;36:109–25.
26. Demirci H, Christianson M. Orbital and adnexal sarcoidosis:analysis of clinical features and systemic disease in 30 cases. Am J Ophthalmol. 2011;151: 1074–80.
27. Prabhakaran VC, Saeed P, Esmaeli B, et al. Orbital and adnexal sarcoidosis. Arch Ophthalmol. 2007;125: 1657–62.
28. Mavrikakis I, Rootman J. Diverse clinical presentations of orbital sarcoid. Am J Ophthalmol. 2007;144: 769–75.
29. Collison JM, Miller NR, Green WR. Involvement of orbital tissues by sarcoid. Am J Ophthalmol. 1986; 102:302–7.
30. Cornblath WT, Elner V, Rolfe M. Extraocular muscle involvement in sarcoidosis. Ophthalmology. 1993; 100:501–5.
31. Patel AS, Kelman SE, Duncan GW, Rismondo V. Painless diplopia caused by extraocular muscle sarcoid. Arch Ophthalmol. 1994;112:879–80.
32. Brooks SE, Sangueza OP, Field RS. Extraocular muscle involvement in sarcoidosis: a clinicopathologic report. J AAPOS. 1997;1:125–8.
33. Patrinely JR, Osborn AG, Anderson RL, Whiting AS. Computed tomographic features of nonthyroid extraocular muscle enlargement. Ophthalmology. 1989;96:1038–47.
34. Kao SC, Rootman J. Unusual orbital presentations of dural sarcoidosis. Can J Ophthalmol. 1996;31: 195–200.
35. Cottin V, Muller-Quernheim J. Sarcoidosis from bench to bedside: a state of the art series for the clinician. Eur Respir J. 2012;40:14–6.
36. Selroos O, Gronhagen-Riska C. Angiotensin converting enzyme. III. Changes in serum level as an indicator of disease activity in untreated sarcoidosis. Scand J Respir Dis. 1979;60:328–36.

37. Tomita H, Sato S, Matsuda R, et al. Serum lysozyme levels and clinical features of sarcoidosis. Lung. 1999;177:161–7.

38. Wj P, Neves RA, Rodriguez A, et al. The value of combined serum angiotensin-converting enzyme and gallium scan in diagnosing ocular sarcoidosis. Ophthalmology. 1995;102:2007–11.

39. Evans M, Sharma O, LaBree L, Smith R, Rao NA. Differences in clinical findings between Caucasians and African Americans with biopsy-proven sarcoidosis. Ophthalmology. 2007;114:325–33.

40. Spaide RF, Ward DL. Conjunctival biopsy in the diagnosis of sarcoidosis. Br J Ophthalmol. 1990;74:469–71.

41. Chung YM, Lin YC, Huang DF, et al. Conjunctival biopsy in sarcoidosis. J Chin Med Assoc. 2006;69:472–7.

42. Leavitt JA, Campbell RJ. Cost-effectiveness in the diagnosis of sarcoidosis: the conjunctival biopsy. Eye. 1998;12:959–62.

43. Peckham DG, Spiteri MA. Sarcoidosis. Postgrad Med J. 1996;72:196–200.

44. Baughman RR, Bradley DA, Lower EE. Infliximab in chronic ocular inflammation. Int J Clin Pharmacol Ther. 2005;43:7–11.

45. Baughman RR, Lower EE, Bradley DA, et al. Etanercept for refractory ocular sarcoidosis. Results of double-blind, randomized trial. Chest. 2005;128:1062–47.

Orbital and Adnexal Sjögren Syndrome

5

Shivani Gupta and Hakan Demirci

Sjögren syndrome (SS) is a chronic, systemic autoimmune disorder in which inflammation of the exocrine glands results in secretory gland dysfunction. This, in turn, leads to dryness of mucosal surfaces with subsequent dry mouth (xerostomia), dry eyes (keratoconjunctivitis sicca), and other extraglandular symptoms [1–3]. When Sjögren syndrome is not present in the context of connective tissue disorders such as scleroderma, rheumatoid arthritis, or systemic lupus erythematosus, it is designated as primary Sjögren syndrome (pSS). When an association exists, it is categorized as secondary Sjögren syndrome (sSS). Varying prevalence rates of SS have been reported, with a range between 0.1 and 4.8 % [4]. The lack of consistent diagnostic criteria used and the varied populations studied likely contribute to this wide range [4]. Although the disease may affect all individuals, middle-aged women are overwhelmingly more commonly affected, with female-male ratio of approximately 9:1 [4, 5].

5.1 Systemic Features

While multiple-organ systems may be involved, the salivary glands and lacrimal glands are more commonly affected, leading to reduced excretory function and the characteristic symptoms of dry mouth and dry eyes. In one series of dry eye patients, 10.9 % of patients had underlying pSS, suggesting that this potential underlying etiology should not be overlooked among dry eye patients [6]. Approximately one third of patients may present with extraglandular symptoms, including involvement of the skin, joints, liver, pancreas, thyroid gland, and hematologic, neurologic, and cardiovascular systems [1, 7]. Musculature may also be affected, leading to fibromyalgia-like symptoms and chronic fatigue [8, 9]. In addition, SS may lead to significant functional disability and reduced health-related quality of life, with affected patients suffering from increased depression, fatigue, and pain [5, 9]. In one study, functional disability in SS patients was seen to be as high as patients with systemic lupus erythematosus, despite comparatively reduced end-organ damage [10]. Furthermore, health care costs for patients with SS may double that of the average primary

S. Gupta, MD, MPH (✉)
Department of Ophthalmology and Visual Science, W.K. Kellogg Eye Center, University of Michigan, 1000 Wall Street, Ann Arbor, MI, 48105, USA

Veterans Administration Ann Arbor Health Care System, Ann Arbor, MI, USA
e-mail: shivanig@med.umich.edu

H. Demirci, MD
Department of Ophthalmology and Visual Science, W.K. Kellogg Eye Center, University of Michigan, Ann Arbor, MI, USA

H. Demirci (ed.), *Orbital Inflammatory Diseases and Their Differential Diagnosis*, Essentials in Ophthalmology, DOI 10.1007/978-3-662-46528-8_5,
© Springer-Verlag Berlin Heidelberg 2015

care patient, compounding the physical and psychosocial effects of this chronic disease [1].

Primary Sjögren syndrome has been associated with cancer, most commonly non-Hodgkin's lymphoma (NHL) [11]. Patients with pSS have a 16–20-fold increased risk of lymphoma, and in one series of 723 consecutive patients with pSS, 1 in 5 deaths was attributable to lymphoma [12–14]. Identified risk factors for development of lymphoma in pSS patients include permanent swelling of major salivary glands, lymphadenopathy, cryoglobulinemia, splenomegaly, low complement levels of C4 and C3, lymphopenia, skin vasculitis or palpable purpura, M-component in serum or urine, peripheral neuropathy, glomerulonephritis, and elevated beta2 microglobulin [14]. Recent studies have also identified associations with genetic factors, CD4 lymphocytopenia, and ectopic germinal center-like structures in minor salivary gland biopsies [14–16]. In a recent Taiwanese population-based study, the incidence of cancer among 7,852 patients with pSS was 2.9 %, with greater incidence among men [11]. In this cohort, only patients aged 25–44 years had an increased risk for cancer compared to same sex-age groups [11]. The study confirmed previously published data regarding the increased risk of NHL but also noted increased risk of multiple myeloma and thyroid cancer among female pSS patients [11].

5.2   Diagnostic Evaluation

The classification of pSS based on the revised American-European Consensus Group criteria (AECG 2002, Table 5.1) combines clinical signs and symptoms with histopathologic and laboratory testing. Four or more of the detailed criteria are required, and these include ocular symptoms, ocular signs, oral symptoms, salivary gland involvement, histopathologic findings, and presence of autoantibodies against the Ro/SSA and La/SSB ribonucleoprotein complexes [7]. Though not a part of the AECG criteria, the presence of positive ANA and RF antibodies may aid in the evaluation of SSA-/SSB-negative patients, as pSS has been shown to occur more commonly in ANA- and RF-positive individuals [17]. More

recently, the American College of Rheumatology proposed a new classification for pSS, requiring two of the following three criteria to be present: (1) positive serum anti-SSA and/or anti-SSB or positive rheumatoid factor and antinuclear antibody titer >1:320, (2) ocular staining score >3, or (3) presence of focal lymphocytic sialoadenitis with a focus score >1 focus/4 mm^2 in labial salivary gland biopsy samples [18]. Although this classification is simpler and based on purely objective parameters, in certain populations it may demonstrate less sensitivity and specificity compared to the AECG and other classification criteria [19]. Given the presence of multiple classification systems as well as heterogeneity in disease manifestations, challenges exist in the standardization of pSS evaluation. Advances in genomics and proteomics may allow for the identification of biomarkers that aid in diagnosis at early stages of disease, before pathologic destruction of exocrine glands occurs, or to identify susceptible individuals prior to disease onset [8]. For example, in one recent study, proteomic evaluation of the tear film was evaluated and proposed as a noninvasive diagnostic test for SS [20]. Others have suggested the use of ultrasonography as a noninvasive tool for the diagnosis of pSS as well as to monitor disease progression and in lieu of more invasive salivary gland testing such as sialography or sialoscintigraphy [21–23].

5.3   Pathogenesis

The underlying etiology of Sjögren syndrome is not clearly elucidated; however, genetic, hormonal, and environmental factors are thought to be involved. As with other autoimmune disorders, extrinsic or intrinsic stimuli in genetically predisposed individuals are thought to be responsible for disease manifestation [4]. Perimenopausal women are more commonly affected by SS, suggesting an immunoregulatory effect of sex hormones on the development of disease, likely related to an imbalance of the estrogen-androgen ratio [3, 24]. Animal models have demonstrated acceleration of pathologic changes including lymphocyte infiltration and apoptosis in genetically

Table 5.1 Revised international classification criteria for Sjögren syndrome [7]

I. Ocular symptoms—a positive response to at least one of the following questions:

(a) Have you had daily, persistent, troublesome dry eyes for more than 3 months? (b) Do you have a recurrent sensation of sand or gravel in the eyes? (c) Do you use tear substitutes more than three times a day?

II. Oral symptoms—a positive response to at least one of the following questions:

(a) Have you had a daily feeling of dry mouth for more than 3 months? (b) Have you had recurrently or persistently swollen salivary glands as an adult? (c) Do you frequently drink liquids to aid in swallowing dry food?

III. Ocular signs—objective evidence of ocular involvement defined as a positive result for at least one of the following tests:

(a) Schirmer test for tear function, performed without anesthesia (positive result ≤5 mm in 5 min). (b) Rose Bengal score or other ocular dye score (positive result score ≥4 on the van Bijsterveld scoring system)

IV. Histopathology—in minor salivary gland (obtained through normal-appearing mucosa) focal lymphocytic sialoadenitis, evaluated by an expert histopathologist, with a focus score of 1 (defined as the number of lymphocytic foci which are adjacent to normal-appearing mucous acini and contain >50 lymphocytes) per 4 mm^2 of glandular tissue)

V. Salivary gland involvement—objective evidence of salivary gland involvement defined by a positive result for at least one of the following tests:

(a) Unstimulated whole salivary flow (<1.5 mL in 15 min). (b) Parotid sialography showing presence of diffuse sialectasis (punctate, cavitary, or destructive pattern) without evidence of obstruction in the major ducts. (c) Salivary scintigraphy showing delayed uptake, reduced concentration, or delayed excretion of tracer

VI. Autoantibodies to Ro/SSA or La/SSB antigens or both

For primary SS

In patients without any potentially associated disease, primary SS may be defined as follows:

(a) The presence of any 4 of the 6 items is indicative of primary SS, as long as either item IV (histopathology) or VI (serology) is positive

(b) The presence of any 3 of the 4 objective criteria items (i.e., items III, IV, V, VI)

(c) The classification tree procedure represents a valid alternative method for classification, although it should be more properly used in clinical-epidemiological survey

For secondary SS

In patients with a potentially associated disease (for instance, another well-defined connective tissue disease), the presence of item I or item II plus any 2 from among items III, IV, and V may be considered as indicative of secondary SS:

Exclusion criteria:

Past head and neck radiation treatment

Hepatitis C infection

Acquired immunodeficiency disease (AIDS)

Preexisting lymphoma

Sarcoidosis

Graft-versus-host disease

Use of anticholinergic drugs (since a time shorter than fourfold the half-life of the drug)

predisposed animals following removal of ovarian sex hormones and conversely prevention following sex hormone replacement [25]. Viral triggers have also been proposed, with activation of immune mechanisms through the type I IFN system, which has been widely implicated in autoimmune disorders [4]. MHC class II genes are associated with pSS, in particular HLA-DR and DQ alleles [3]. Polymorphisms of the IRF-5 and STAT4 genes, as well as the increase in copy of immunoregulatory genes FCGRB and CCL3L1, may increase disease susceptibility [4, 26–30]. Autoantibody production including anti-SSA/Ro and anti-La/SSB La is associated with early onset and longer duration of disease, as well as more intense immune cell infiltration, higher frequency of extraglandular manifestation, and parotid gland enlargement [3].

5.4   Histopathologic Features

The underlying histopathology of SS includes periductal lymphocytic infiltration of salivary and lacrimal glands and destruction of tissues [31]. Infiltrates generally consist of CD4+ T cells, CD8+ T cells, B cells, and macrophages [8]. While the majority of the infiltrating cell population is comprised of T cells, B cell autoreactivity is thought to play an important role in both preclinical and clinical disease [8, 25]. Apoptosis of acinar cells is also a prominent feature, leading to hypofunction and hyposecretion of fluids, and in animal studies has been shown to occur after immune cell infiltration following oophorectomy [25]. There continues to remain some debate as to whether apoptosis follows the inflammatory phase, and some authors suggest that apoptosis may have a role in initiating the disease process in genetically susceptible individuals [24]. Non-apoptotic mechanisms may also play a role, leading to hypofunction of secretory mechanisms. These include neural dysregulation via inhibition of neurotransmitter release by cytokines, increased levels of cholinesterase leading to reduced Ach, and M3R antimuscarinic antibody blockade [8, 24]. Changes in the expression and distribution of aquaporin5 in the acini of salivary glands are thought to contribute to reduced fluid secretion, both in the inflammatory and noninflammatory phases [24].

5.5   Ocular Manifestations and Management of Primary Sjögren Syndrome

Tears are crucial for the maintenance of a healthy ocular surface. Not only do they provide lubrication but contain a host of growth factors, vitamins, and neuropeptides that promote a healthy environment for the ocular surface epithelium [32]. Ocular signs and symptoms related to pSS are a result of immune cell infiltration and destruction of the lacrimal gland, leading to aqueous tear deficiency and the secondary effects of this, sicca syndrome. Patients may complain of dryness, foreign body sensation, redness, fatigue,

itching, reduction in vision, and reflex tearing. Deficiency of tears also leads to a proinflammatory response, immune cell infiltration, loss of surface epithelial integrity, and eventually keratinization of the ocular surface [33]. This latter process is known as squamous metaplasia. In addition, meibomian gland dropout may occur and lead to increased tear evaporation, compounding the effect of reduced tear production and leading to increased fluorescein and rose Bengal staining that is seen in SS-related ATD (aqueous tear deficiency) vs. non-SS ATD [34, 35]. In severe cases, persistent corneal epithelial defects or ulceration may also occur, putting patients at risk for corneal infection.

Evaluation for ocular involvement in SS begins with a patient history focused on symptoms of dry eye mentioned previously, as well as use of artificial tear substitutes and their effect on alleviating symptoms. Formal scales such as Ocular Surface Disease Index (OSDI) and OCI patient symptom questionnaires may be used. Ophthalmic testing includes Schirmer basal tear secretion testing, evaluation of tear film height, rose Bengal staining and score, fluorescein staining, lissamine green staining, tear breakup time evaluation, assessment of meibomian gland dysfunction, and careful conjunctival and corneal examination to assess for punctate epithelial erosions, corneal filaments, epithelial defects, corneal thinning, ulceration, or squamous metaplasia. Lacrimal scintigraphy is another tool that has been evaluated in SS patients and been shown to correlate closely with rose Bengal staining, Schirmer testing, tear breakup time, and the ocular surface disease index [36]. Other specialized tests may include tear osmolarity testing, tear lactoferrin and lysozyme measurement, and impression cytology for evaluation of goblet cells. More recently, in vivo confocal microscopy of the lacrimal gland has been shown to demonstrate acinar unit dilatation, interstitial fibrosis, and inflammatory cells in SS patients and may aid in the noninvasive evaluation of SS patients [37].

A wide array of treatments have been studied for the management of dry eyes in SS patients including topical lubricants, autologous serum, topical corticosteroids, topical anti-inflammatory therapy, secretagogues, and systemic immuno-suppressive agents, as well as interventions such as punctual occlusion with plugs or cautery [38].

Initial treatment strategies for aqueous deficiency in SS begin with aqueous supplementation, generally using artificial tear substitutes, which show consistent improvement in symptoms over baseline [38]. These vary from drops to more viscous gels and ointments. Studies suggest that the use of more viscous lubricants affords greater comfort with reduced frequency of use and increased duration of effect [39]. The use of serum tears has been advocated in the treatment of dye eyes and ocular surface disease due to the presence of growth factors and bactericidal agents, which provide additional benefits to aqueous supplementation in maintaining a healthy ocular surface epithelium [32]. It has been shown, when diluted with saline, to improve both subjective and objective dry eye parameters among SS patients [40].

When aqueous supplementation is insufficient to control sicca symptoms, reduction in tear drainage may be addressed. This can be done via placement of punctual plugs to mechanically occlude one or both puncta on each side or thermal punctual cautery. Placement of Smartplugs in the inferior canaliculi only has been shown to improve Schirmer I testing as well as reduce tear breakup time [41]. Additionally, partial cauterization of the puncta to achieve a punctual opening of 0.5 mm improves clinical signs such as fluorescein staining, rose Bengal staining, tear breakup time, and Schirmer I testing, an effect that is sustained for up to 2 years following treatment [42]. The use of topical anti-inflammatory agents has also been prospectively studied, including corticosteroids and nonsteroidal anti-inflammatory drugs [38]. While varying improvement in subjective and objective parameters has been shown, side effects such as increased intraocular pressure, cataract formation, and corneal epithelial staining may limit their use long term. Topical cyclosporine, in varying concentrations, has been shown in several prospective, randomized controlled trials to improve ocular signs such as surface staining, Schirmer testing, and tear breakup time as well [38]. In one study, a reduction of activated lymphocytes was noted in conjunctival biopsies of SS patients treated with 6 months of topical 0.05 % cyclosporine [43]. Given its relative clinical safety with long-term use, it use should be considered in patients with SS [38].

As described in a recent review of 66 previously published reports regarding the treatment of SS-associated dry eyes, several oral agents have been studied including secretagogues such as pilocarpine and cevimeline [38]. The use of oral pilocarpine has been shown to improve sicca symptoms in SS patients, and in one study of 5 mg twice daily, it showed significantly better subjective outcomes and improved rose Bengal staining compared with artificial tear use or punctual occlusion [44]. In another study, tear meniscus height as measured by Visante OCT was shown to improve following oral administration of pilocarpine, 5 mg twice daily, as were signs and symptoms of dry eye [45]. Cevimeline has also shown promising results in double-blinded, randomized controlled trials, with recommended dosage of 30 mg three times per day [38]. A number of other systemic agents have been studied, including corticosteroids, cyclosporine, hydroxychloroquine, rituximab, infliximab, etanercept, mycophenolic acid, and interferon alpha-2. Although these agents may be beneficial in the treatment of systemic manifestations of SS and for the treatment of SS-associated dry eyes, there is insufficient data to suggest significant improvement with their use [38].

Compliance with Ethical Requirements Shivani Gupta and Hakan Demirci declare that they have no conflict of interest. No human studies were carried out by the authors for this article. No animal studies were carried out by the authors for this article.

References

1. Ramos-Casals M, et al. Primary Sjogren syndrome. BMJ. 2012;344:e3821.
2. Ramos-Casals MFJ. Primary Sjögren's syndrome. In: Hellmann D, Imboden J, Stone J, editors. Current diagnosis and treatment in rheumatology. New York: McGraw-Hill; 2007. p. 237–45.
3. Yamamoto K. Pathogenesis of Sjögren's syndrome. Autoimmun Rev. 2003;2(1):13–8.

4. Mavragani CP, Moutsopoulos HM. The geoepidemiology of Sjogren's syndrome. Autoimmun Rev. 2010;9(5):A305–10.
5. Segal B, et al. Primary Sjogren's syndrome: health experiences and predictors of health quality among patients in the United States. Health Qual Life Outcomes. 2009;7:46.
6. Akpek EK, et al. Evaluation of patients with dry eye for presence of underlying Sjogren syndrome. Cornea. 2009;28(5):493–7.
7. Vitali C, et al. Classification criteria for Sjogren's syndrome: a revised version of the European criteria proposed by the American-European Consensus Group. Ann Rheum Dis. 2002;61(6):554–8.
8. Nguyen CQ, Peck AB. Unraveling the pathophysiology of Sjogren syndrome-associated dry eye disease. Ocul Surf. 2009;7(1):11–27.
9. Hackett KL, et al. Impaired functional status in primary Sjogren's syndrome. Arthritis Care Res (Hoboken). 2012;64(11):1760–4.
10. Sutcliffe N, et al. Functional disability and end organ damage in patients with systemic lupus erythematosus (SLE), SLE and Sjogren's syndrome (SS), and primary SS. J Rheumatol. 1998;25(1):63–8.
11. Weng MY, et al. Incidence of cancer in a nationwide population cohort of 7852 patients with primary Sjogren's syndrome in Taiwan. Ann Rheum Dis. 2012;71(4):524–7.
12. Ioannidis JP, Vassiliou VA, Moutsopoulos HM. Long-term risk of mortality and lymphoproliferative disease and predictive classification of primary Sjogren's syndrome. Arthritis Rheum. 2002;46(3):741–7.
13. Solans-Laque R, et al. Risk, predictors, and clinical characteristics of lymphoma development in primary Sjogren's syndrome. Semin Arthritis Rheum. 2011; 41(3):415–23.
14. Jonsson MV, Theander E, Jonsson R. Predictors for the development of non-Hodgkin lymphoma in primary Sjogren's syndrome. Presse Med. 2012;41(9 Pt 2):e511–6.
15. Theander E, et al. Lymphoid organisation in labial salivary gland biopsies is a possible predictor for the development of malignant lymphoma in primary Sjogren's syndrome. Ann Rheum Dis. 2011;70(8): 1363–8.
16. Ismail F, et al. Primary Sjogren's syndrome and B-non-Hodgkin lymphoma: role of CD4+ T lymphocytopenia. Rheumatol Int. 2013;33:1021–5.
17. Liew MS, et al. Prevalence and predictors of Sjogren's syndrome in a prospective cohort of patients with aqueous-deficient dry eye. Br J Ophthalmol. 2012; 96(12):1498–503.
18. Shiboski SC, et al. American College of Rheumatology classification criteria for Sjogren's syndrome: a data-driven, expert consensus approach in the Sjogren's International Collaborative Clinical Alliance cohort. Arthritis Care Res (Hoboken). 2012;64(4):475–87.
19. Tsuboi H, et al. Validation of different sets of criteria for the diagnosis of Sjogren's syndrome in Japanese patients. Mod Rheumatol. 2013;23(2):219–25.
20. Tomosugi N, et al. Diagnostic potential of tear proteomic patterns in Sjogren's syndrome. J Proteome Res. 2005;4(3):820–5.
21. Cornec D, et al. Contribution of salivary gland ultrasonography to the diagnosis of Sjogren's syndrome: toward new diagnostic criteria? Arthritis Rheum. 2013;65(1):216–25.
22. Takagi Y, et al. Salivary gland ultrasonography: can it be an alternative to sialography as an imaging modality for Sjogren's syndrome? Ann Rheum Dis. 2010;69(7):1321–4.
23. Milic V, et al. Ultrasonography of major salivary glands could be an alternative tool to sialoscintigraphy in the American-European classification criteria for primary Sjogren's syndrome. Rheumatology (Oxford). 2012;51(6):1081–5.
24. Hayashi T. Dysfunction of lacrimal and salivary glands in Sjogren's syndrome: nonimmunologic injury in preinflammatory phase and mouse model. J Biomed Biotechnol. 2011;2011:407031.
25. Mostafa S, Seamon V, Azzarolo AM. Influence of sex hormones and genetic predisposition in Sjogren's syndrome: a new clue to the immunopathogenesis of dry eye disease. Exp Eye Res. 2012;96(1):88–97.
26. Miceli-Richard C, et al. Association of an IRF5 gene functional polymorphism with Sjogren's syndrome. Arthritis Rheum. 2007;56(12):3989–94.
27. Miceli-Richard C, et al. The CGGGG insertion/deletion polymorphism of the IRF5 promoter is a strong risk factor for primary Sjogren's syndrome. Arthritis Rheum. 2009;60(7):1991–7.
28. Korman BD, et al. Variant form of STAT4 is associated with primary Sjogren's syndrome. Genes Immun. 2008;9(3):267–70.
29. Nordmark G, et al. Additive effects of the major risk alleles of IRF5 and STAT4 in primary Sjogren's syndrome. Genes Immun. 2009;10(1):68–76.
30. Mamtani M, et al. Association of copy number variation in the FCGR3B gene with risk of autoimmune diseases. Genes Immun. 2010;11(2):155–60.
31. Moriyama M, et al. Cytokine/chemokine profiles contribute to understanding the pathogenesis and diagnosis of primary Sjogren's syndrome. Clin Exp Immunol. 2012;169(1):17–26.
32. Quinto GG, Campos M, Behrens A. Autologous serum for ocular surface diseases. Arq Bras Oftalmol. 2008;71(6 Suppl):47–54.
33. Zhou D, et al. Critical involvement of macrophage infiltration in the development of Sjogren's syndrome-associated dry eye. Am J Pathol. 2012;181(3):753–60.
34. Shimazaki J, et al. Meibomian gland dysfunction in patients with Sjogren syndrome. Ophthalmology. 1998;105(8):1485–8.
35. Goto E, et al. Tear evaporation rates in Sjogren syndrome and non-Sjogren dry eye patients. Am J Ophthalmol. 2007;144(1):81–5.
36. Erhamamci S, et al. The clinical value and histopathological correlation of lacrimal scintigraphy in patients with primary Sjogren's syndrome. Nucl Med Commun. 2012;33(7):689–94.

37. Sato EA, et al. Lacrimal gland in Sjogren's syndrome. Ophthalmology. 2010;117(5):1055–1055 e3.
38. Akpek EK, et al. Treatment of Sjogren's syndrome-associated dry eye an evidence-based review. Ophthalmology. 2011;118(7):1242–52.
39. Bhojwani R, et al. Treatment of dry eye: an analysis of the British Sjogren's syndrome association comparing substitute tear viscosity and subjective efficacy. Cont Lens Anterior Eye. 2011;34(6):269–73.
40. Tsubota K, et al. Treatment of dry eye by autologous serum application in Sjogren's syndrome. Br J Ophthalmol. 1999;83(4):390–5.
41. Egrilmez S, et al. Clinical efficacy of the SmartPlug in the treatment of primary Sjogren's syndrome with keratoconjunctivitis sicca: one-year follow-up study. Rheumatol Int. 2011;31(12):1567–70.
42. Holzchuh R, et al. Two-year outcome of partial lacrimal punctal occlusion in the management of dry eye related to Sjogren syndrome. Curr Eye Res. 2011;36(6):507–12.
43. Kunert KS, Tisdale AS, Stern ME, Smith JA, Gipson IK. Analysis of topical cyclosporine treatment of patients with dry eye syndrome: effect on conjunctival lymphocytes. Arch Ophthalmol. 2000;118(11):1489–96.
44. Tsifetaki N, et al. Oral pilocarpine for the treatment of ocular symptoms in patients with Sjogren's syndrome: a randomised 12 week controlled study. Ann Rheum Dis. 2003;62(12):1204–7.
45. Ibrahim OM, et al. Visante optical coherence tomography and tear function test evaluation of cholinergic treatment response in patients with Sjogren syndrome. Cornea. 2013;32:653–7.

Antineutrophil Cytoplasmic Antibody (ANCA)-Associated Vasculitic Orbital Syndromes

6

Gangadhara Sundar

6.1 Introduction

Orbital inflammatory disorders are the most common type of orbital disease and may be either of infectious or noninfectious etiology. Noninfectious orbital inflammatory disorders may be further classified into those of specific and nonspecific etiology. As a general rule, all noninfectious inflammatory disorders are specific until proven otherwise (Fig. 6.1). Almost all noninfectious specific orbital inflammatory disorders are proposed to be of autoimmune etiology with variable combination of both cell-mediated and immune complex-mediated mechanisms contributing to the various manifestations of the disease.

Autoimmune vasculitides comprise a major proportion of autoimmune specific orbital inflammatory disorders. This diverse group of orbital and systemic disorders is characterized by an angiocentric inflammation resulting in perivascular and vascular infiltration of either the small, intermediate, or large vessels with resultant consequences of significant morbidity or even mortality, if untreated. An antigenic stimulus may result in an abnormal immune response with immune complex formation, triggering an immunological cascade with resultant inflammation, vascular infiltration, and tissue destruction.

The three major categories of systemic vasculitides are large vessel vasculitis (chronic granulomatous arteritis) e.g., giant cell arteritis, medium-sized vessel vasculitis (necrotizing arteritis) e.g., polyarteritis nodosa, and small vessel vasculitis (necrotizing polyangiitis), e.g., GPA (Wegener's) (Fig. 6.2) [1]. Clinical manifestations in these patients are similar to nonspecific orbital inflammatory syndrome. Thus a high degree of clinical suspicion, with appropriate laboratory workup, and, in specific cases, a tissue diagnosis are what help make a definitive diagnosis. This in turn helps direct specific management before significant morbidity and even mortality may ensue.

Eighty to ninety percent of small vessel vasculitides are associated with the presence of antineutrophil cytoplasmic antibody (ANCA), termed ANCA-associated vasculitis (AAV) or ANCA disease [2]. These include granulomatosis with polyangiitis (GPA), formerly known as Wegener's granulomatosis, microscopic polyangiitis (MPA), and the allergic granulomatosis with polyangiitis (AGPA) formerly known as Churg-Strauss syndrome [3]. These new terminologies were recommended by the boards of the American Society of Nephrology, the American College of Rheumatology and the EULAR which urged a shift from eponyms to disease-descriptive or cause-based nomenclature. The AAVs are distin-

G. Sundar, DO, FRCSEd, FAMS
Department of Ophthalmology, Orbit and Oculofacial Surgery, Singapore, Singapore

Adjunct Faculty, Department of Pediatrics, National University Hospital, Singapore, Singapore
e-mail: gangadhara_sundar@nuhs.edu.sg; gsundar1@yahoo.com

H. Demirci (ed.), *Orbital Inflammatory Diseases and Their Differential Diagnosis*, Essentials in Ophthalmology, DOI 10.1007/978-3-662-46528-8_6,
© Springer-Verlag Berlin Heidelberg 2015

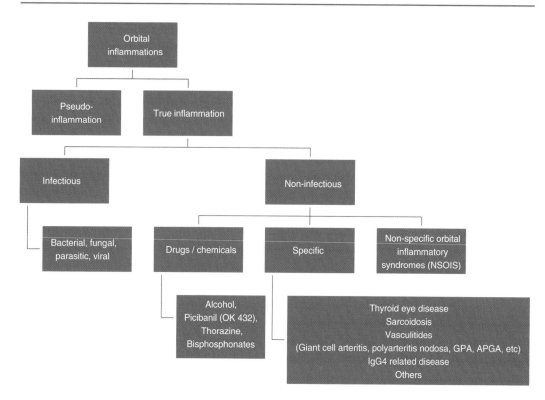

Fig. 6.1 Practical classification of orbital inflammatory diseases

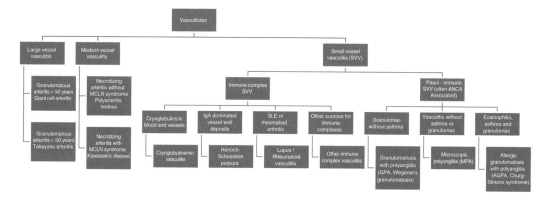

Fig. 6.2 Classification of vasculitic disorders

guished from other systemic small vessel vasculitides by the absence of immune deposits. Of interest to the ophthalmologist are the granulomatosis with polyangiitis (GPA) and allergic granulomatosis with polyangiitis (AGPA), both of which shall be addressed in this chapter. Although grouped together, AGPA has a different presentation and prognosis compared with the other ANCA-associated vasculitides.

Antineutrophil cytoplasmic antibodies were described in 1982 [4] and associated with Wegener's granulomatosis in 1985 [5]. Two types of assays in common use are immunofluorescence (IF) and enzyme immunoassay (EIA). By immunofluorescence, 3 distinct types of ANCA have been described: cytoplasmic (c-ANCA), perinuclear (p-ANCA), and atypical (x- or a-ANCA). In patients with vasculitis, the c-ANCA

Fig. 6.3 Giant cell and granuloma formation in vasculitic disorders

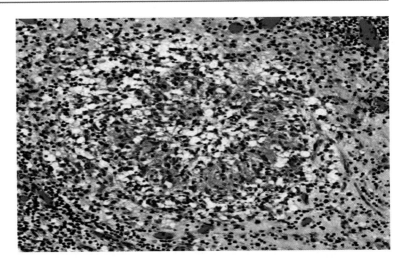

pattern is associated with the presence of protein-ase-3 antibodies known as PR-3 ANCA.

In the early phases, polymorphonuclear cellular infiltration occurs, followed by lymphocytic, plasma cellular, and monocytic infiltration as the disease progresses. Subsequent fibrinoid deposition, necrosis, and endothelial damage result in stenosis and thrombosis with clinical manifestations of ischemia and tissue necrosis. In specific conditions like GPA and giant cell arteritis, giant cell and granuloma formation also occurs (Fig. 6.3).

GPA has necrotizing granulomatous inflammation superimposed on the vasculitis. AGPA has adult-onset asthma, allergic rhinitis, eosinophilia, and granulomatous inflammation in addition to vasculitis. MPA has only the vasculitis, without granulomatous inflammation, asthma, or eosinophilia. The clinical manifestations of the above conditions are protean and can affect many different organs individually (limited form of disease) or in combination (disseminated disease).

6.2   Granulomatosis with Polyangiitis (GPA, Wegener's Granulomatosis)

Granulomatosis with polyangiitis (Wegener's) is a multiorgan system disease of unknown etiology characterized by granulomatous inflammation, tissue necrosis, and variable degrees of vasculitis in small- and medium-sized blood vessels. Although initially described by Klinger in 1931 [6], it was recognized as a definitive entity after Friedrich Wegener reported three patients in 1939 [7].

GPA is a disease of unknown etiology primarily involving the upper and lower respiratory tracts and the kidneys, which, if untreated, has major organ- and life-threatening consequences. The incidence is estimated to be four to eight per million population [8] with prevalence estimated to be 30 per million population in the United States [9]. Typically seen in Caucasian men in the fourth to fifth decade, without any specific gender predilection, it may present as a classic disseminated or rarely in the limited form. The limited form of the disease is more commonly seen in women [10] and in Asians. Less than 15 % of the disease is seen in children. It may present either to the general physician or to the ophthalmologist with acute to subacute symptoms either partially or completely unresponsive to conventional and symptomatic management. In most cases, antineutrophil cytoplasmic antibodies (ANCAs) against proteinase-3 (PR-3) [11] are thought to result in neutrophilic and eosinophilic vascular and perivascular infiltration with resultant narrowing, ischemia, and damage of the organs affected [12]. The clinical spectrum of organ systems involved in GPA is summarized in Fig. 6.4. Classic disseminated GPA, characterized by a triad of upper and lower respiratory tract involvement and glomerulonephritis, may present either

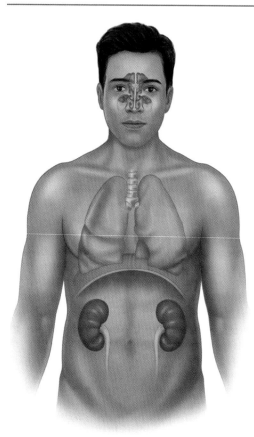

Table 6.1 Granulomatosis with polyangiitis (GPA, Wegener's granulomatosis) presentation

Disseminated disease	Limited disease
Acute disease, easier, earlier diagnosis	Insidious or subacute disease, difficult or late diagnosis, more common in women
Lab tests positive, histopathology – typical	Lab tests may be negative Histopathology – atypical

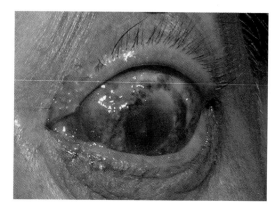

Fig. 6.5 Necrotizing scleritis presentation in GPA (Wegener's)

Fig. 6.4 Clinical spectrum of organ systems involved in GPA

as an acute rapidly progressive disease or rarely a chronic disease. Upper respiratory tract involvement is manifested by sinusitis, epistaxis, and nasal bone destruction with adjacent orbital involvement. Lower respiratory tract involvement is manifested by respiratory tract ulceration and pneumonitis. Renal failure from rapidly progressive glomerulonephritis is not uncommon in untreated cases. Extrapulmonary lesions may affect the skin, joint, heart, and the eyes.

A limited form is commonly seen in females with a less severe clinical course associated with upper and lower respiratory system involved, thus resulting in delayed or missed diagnosis [13]. Significant differences between the acute, systemic form and an insidious limited form of the disease are shown in Table 6.1.

Ophthalmic involvement is seen in about 50 % of all cases. Ocular manifestations are frequently bilateral and may be protean, thus making diagno-

sis difficult with delayed and resultant morbidity, especially when clinical suspicion is low. Left untreated, potential blinding complications include severe necrotizing scleritis (Fig. 6.5), peripheral ulcerative keratitis with corneal perforation [14], retinal vasculitis resulting in retinal arterial occlusion, and orbital inflammatory mass with optic nerve ischemia. Orbital involvement may be either primary [15–21] or more commonly as a result of disease spread from the adjacent paranasal sinuses (Fig. 6.6a,b) or nasopharynx. Rarely fibrotic changes as a result of chronic inflammation may result in socket contracture and enophthalmos (Fig. 6.7) [22]. In fact, owing to the involvement of the nasolacrimal duct drainage pathway secondary to nasal obstruction, it is one of the very few orbital inflammatory diseases that may present as a wet, rather than a dry eye. Common ocular and ocular adnexal manifestations are summarized in Table 6.2 (see also Fig. 6.8). Owing to the severe nature of the disease, the clinical morbidity, and potential mortality, every ophthalmologist should be aware of both the typical and atypical presentations of the disease. Given the protean manifestations,

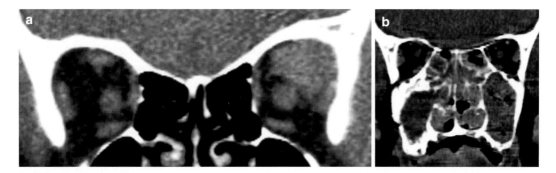

Fig. 6.6 Coronal CT scan showing (**a**) left sided orbital infiltration, (**b**) extensive paranasal sinus involvement with bone destruction and remodeling

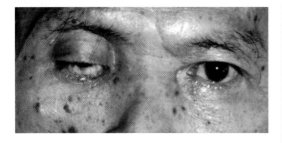

Fig. 6.7 Severe contracted socket in burnt-out disease

Table 6.2 Ophthalmic manifestations of granulomatosis with polyangiitis [23–25]

Ocular manifestations	Ocular adnexal manifestations
Conjunctivitis	Orbital inflammatory syndrome
Peripheral ulcerative keratitis (PUK)	Orbital apex syndrome (Tolosa-Hunt syndrome)
Episcleritis necrotizing scleritis	Dacryoadenitis
Uveitis	Myositis
Retinal vasculitis with vascular occlusion	NLD obstruction/chronic dacryocystitis
	Eyelid granulomas
	Florid xanthelasmas – yellow eyelid sign (Fig. 6.8)
	Optic neuropathy
	Contracted socket with enophthalmos

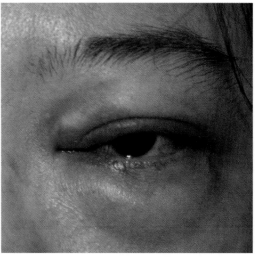

Fig. 6.8 Yellow eyelid sign in limited granulomatosis with polyangiitis (Wegener's)

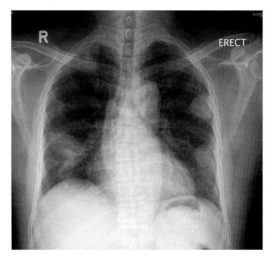

Fig. 6.9 Pulmonary infiltrates characteristic of lower respiratory tract involvement

a high degree of suspicion should be maintained in all patients with any of the clinical presentations shown above especially when bilateral and in the right age group. These include prior or concomitant history of nose/sinus/ENT disorder, upper or lower respiratory ailment (Fig. 6.9), partial response to conventional management, and rapidly progressive and debilitating disease [26].

Appropriate laboratory testing (Table 6.3) should be ordered when the clinical suspicion is present, and when possible, a definitive tissue biopsy should be performed. The presence of two or more of the following criteria is associated with a sensitivity of 88.2 % and a specificity of 92 % [27]:

- Abnormal urinary sediment (red cell casts or >5 RBCs per high-power field)
- Abnormal findings on chest radiograph (nodules, cavities, fixed infiltrates)
- Oral ulcers or nasal discharge
- Granulomatous inflammation on biopsy (Fig. 6.10)

Differential diagnosis depends upon whether the clinical presentation is either acute, typical and disseminated, insidious or a limited form of the disease. Systemic clinical features that help differentiate GPA from AGPA are shown in Table 6.4. In general, the differential diagnosis of vasculitic conditions associated with granulomatous inflammation includes giant cell arteritis, Takayasu's arteritis, Cogan's syndrome, primary angiitis of the CNS, Buerger's disease, and rheumatoid vasculitis.

Management of GPA is challenging, yet rewarding, if a proper assessment of the patient is made followed by a basic understanding of the underlying immunopathogenetic process, which is then used to tailor the treatment to the individual patient. The treatment plan should be based primarily on the stage of the disease and the activity of the disease. The three stages of the disease are an acute, generalized systemic disease which is often severe, a subacute localized form of disease, and finally a chronic indolent or refractory disease. Historically GPA in general had a fatal outcome prior to the advent of immunosuppressive therapy [28], but with the advent of glucocorticoids alone, the median survival increased to 5 months. The introduction of the Fauci and Wolf's NIH standard regimen in the 1970s, combination of glucocorticoids with cyclophosphamide (CYC), further increased the median survival to more than 20 years [29]. However, the substantial long-term toxicity from the above regimen has led to the introduction of less toxic drugs such as methotrexate, azathioprine, or leflunomide, which have better tolerated and manageable side effects. In recent years, newer treatment modalities with biologics such as B-cell blockade and TNF alpha antagonists have also been used.

Table 6.3 Laboratory findings

Nonspecific	Specific
Anemia	c-ANCA
Leukocytosis	Proteinase-3 antibody (Anti PR-3, PR-3 ANCA)
Thrombocytosis	Histopathological diagnosis
Raised ESR, CRP	
Hematuria – microscopic	
Rheumatoid factor (30 % of pts)	

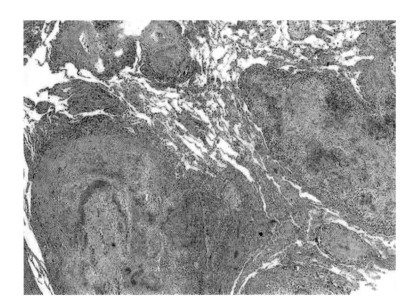

Fig. 6.10 Granulomatous inflammation on biopsy

Table 6.4 Distinguishing diagnostic features of ANCA-associated vasculitis

Feature	GPA	AGPA	Comments
Glomerulonephritis	+++	+	Progressive renal failure uncommon in AGPA
Pulmonary nodules/infiltrates	+++	+++	Asthma and eosinophilia (AGPA)
Upper airway disease	+++	++	ENT disease (GPA)
Skin, purpura	+	++	
Peripheral nerve involvement	++	+++	Prominent feature in GPA
CNS involvement	+	+	

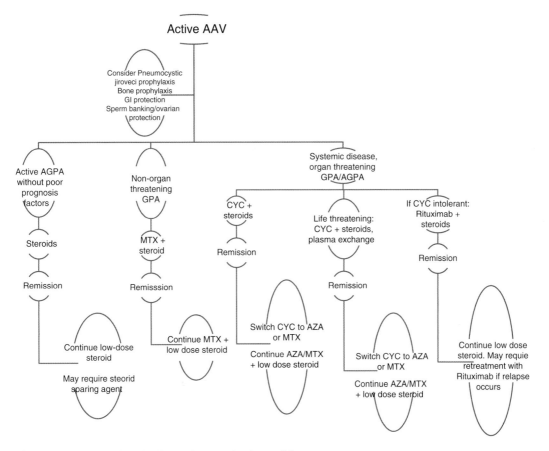

Fig. 6.11 Treatment algorithm for ANCA-associated vasculitis

As a general principle, the first step of the treatment is to induce remission of the active disease, followed by a less aggressive therapy to maintain remission. The final challenge is in the management of the refractory disease state. A treatment algorithm for ANCA-associated vasculitis is depicted in Fig. 6.11. The treatment of choice for severe generalized disease is a combination of glucocorticoids (oral prednisone 1 mg/kg/day or IV methyl prednisolone 500–1,000 mg/day for 3 days for life-threatening disease) and cyclophosphamide (2 mg/kg/day PO or 15–20 mg/kg IV every 3rd week). Given the high cumulative toxicity of cyclophosphamide, treatment may be switched to less toxic agents such as methotrexate (MTX), azathioprine (AZA), or mycophenolate mofetil (MMF) as soon as remission is accomplished. Trimethoprim/sulfamethoxazole may be considered as an alternative for localized disease. Commonly used medications, their indications,

Table 6.5 Dosages and drugs for various stages of GPA (Wegener's)

For induction of remission	Indication	Route/dosage
Cyclophosphamide	Generalized, severe disease	Oral: 2 mg/kg/day
		IV: 15–20 mg/kg q 3 weeks
Methotrexate	Early systemic disease	0.3 mg/kg/week
		IV/SC/PO
Trimethoprim/sulfamethoxazole	Localized disease	2×960 mg/day PO
Plasmapheresis	Severe life-threatening refractory disease	40–60 ml/kg (4–7 cycles)

and dosages are highlighted in Table 6.5. In the 10 % of cases where there is no response to standard treatment, additional therapy with biologic agents, plasmapheresis, or alternative treatments such as deoxyspergualin may be considered.

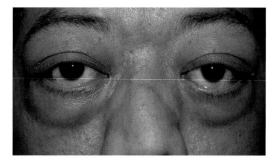

Fig. 6.12 Middle-aged male with bilateral proptosis, asthma, rhinosinusitis, and midline nasal destruction

6.3 Allergic Granulomatosis with Polyangiitis (AGPA, Churg-Strauss Syndrome)

First described by Churg and Strauss in 1951 [30], it is a rare disorder characterized by three salient histopathological features: necrotizing vasculitis, eosinophilic infiltration of tissues, and extravascular granulomata. Other features to supplement a clinical diagnosis include asthma or allergic rhinosinusitis, peak eosinophil count greater than 1,500 cells/ml, and systemic vasculitis involving one or more organs [31]. The mean age of presentation is approximately 50 years with a slight male preponderance.

The etiopathogenesis of AGPA is quite unclear, but a strong association with allergy and atopic disorders including allergic rhinitis, nasal polyposis, and asthma has been noted. Approximately 70 % of patients have elevated IgE levels along with peripheral and tissue eosinophilia. While ANCA may be negative in 60 % of patients, some patients demonstrate ANCA positivity, especially to myeloperoxidase (MPO). When ANCA is present, it is associated with a higher incidence of pulmonary hemorrhage, mononeuritis multiplex, and renal disease [32]. AGPA may be characterized by three distinctive clinical phases. A prodromal allergic phase may begin in late childhood or adulthood which may be present for months to years. This is followed by an eosinophilic infiltration phase with granulomatous inflammation when systemic and orbital features are present. The final third phase is a vasculitic phase with involvement of the small vessels of the eyes and other organ systems [31].

Ophthalmic manifestations are varied and result from granulomatous inflammation, vasculitis, or both. Anterior segment involvement can present as chronic conjunctivitis, conjunctival granulomas, episcleritis, scleritis, or keratouveitis. Orbital infiltration commonly presents as proptosis, although not vision threatening (Fig. 6.12). Neuro-ophthalmic manifestations include cranial neuropathies, amaurotic episodes, and arteritic ischemic optic neuropathy [33]. Vascular involvement may present as a central or branch retinal artery occlusion. Systemic features include pulmonary infiltrate and effusions, alveolar hemorrhage, peripheral neuropathy (mononeuritis multiplex), and involvement of the CNS, lower urinary tract, heart, and gastrointestinal tract. The presence of four or more of the following criteria has a sensitivity of 85 % and a specificity of 99.7 % [34]:

• Asthma
• Peripheral eosinophilia greater than 10 %
• Mononeuropathy or polyneuropathy
• Nonfixed pulmonary infiltrates on chest x-ray
• Paranasal sinus abnormality (Fig. 6.13a,b)
• Biopsy containing a blood vessel with extravascular eosinophils (Fig. 6.14)

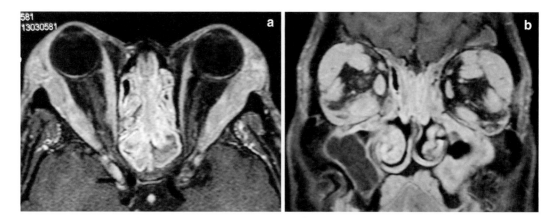

Fig. 6.13 MRI axial (**a**) and coronal (**b**) demonstrating involvement of the extraocular muscles, lacrimal gland, and paranasal sinuses

Fig. 6.14 Biopsy containing a blood vessel with extravascular eosinophils

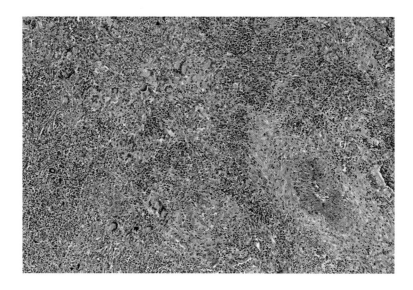

Features associated with a poorer prognosis include creatinemia (>140 mmol/L (1.58 mg/dL)), proteinuria (>1 g/day), or CNS, gastrointestinal, or myocardial involvement [35].

An overview of differences in clinical and laboratory features between AGPA and GPA is shown in Table 6.4.

Most patients may benefit from short course of oral or intravenous corticosteroids to achieve disease remission, especially if not life-threatening. Chronic disease may require long-term low-dose steroids or the use of other steroid-sparing agents. Severe life-threatening disease, although uncommon, may require aggressive management similar to GPA. A conceptual approach to the management of AGPA is shown in Fig. 6.11.

6.4   Summary

The natural history of untreated AAV is rapidly progressive and usually fatal, with a 2-year mortality rate of 85 %. The introduction of cyclophosphamide-based regimens to treat AAV in the 1970s has dramatically reversed patient survival, now at 80 % at 5 years [36]. The aim of treatment is to induce and then maintain disease remission and prevent relapse, using agents with the least adverse event profile. Treatment is tailored according to the disease severity at presentation with more aggressive immunosuppression in the presence of organ-threatening and life-threatening disease [37].

Great advances have occurred in the understanding or the causes and pathogenetic mechanisms underlying AAV over the past 20 years. Mortality rates have been substantially reduced and in fact reversed since the introduction of cyclophosphamide and other alternative immunosuppressant medications in combination with glucocorticoid therapy. However, while mortality has been reduced, chronic relapsing disease, without the offer of cure, poses a great challenge. While rituximab and other biologics hold promise, their cost, toxicity, and lack of long-term evidence make the management of this group of disease challenging.

Acknowledgement Dr Seet JE, Dept of Pathology, National University Hospital, Singapore for the histopathology images.

Compliance with Ethical Requirements Dr JK Gangadhara Sundar declares no conflict of interest.

No human or animal studies were carried out for this article.

References

1. Jennette JC, Falk RJ. Necrotizing arteritis and small vessel vasculitis. Chapter 65. In: Rose NR, Mackay IR, editors. The autoimmune disease. 2006. p. 899–920. ISBN-13:978-0-12-595961-2 ISBN −10: 0-12-595961-3.
2. Falk RJ, Jennette JC. ANCA disease: where is this field heading? J Am Soc Nephrol. 2010;21:745–52.
3. Jennette JC, Falk RJ, Andrassy K, et al. Nomenclature of systemic vasculitides. Proposal of an international consensus conference. Arthritis Rheum. 1994;37:187.
4. Davies D, Moran J, et al. Segmental necrotizing glomerulonephritis with antineutrophil antibody: possible arbovirus aetiology. Br Med J. 1982;285:606.
5. Van der Woude F, Rasmussen N, Lobatto S, et al. Autoantibodies against neutrophils and monocytes: tools for diagnosis and marker of disease activity in Wegener's granulomatosis. Lancet. 1985;1:425–9.
6. Klinger H. Grenzformen der periarteritis nodosa. Frankfurt Z Pathol. 1931;42:455–80.
7. Wegener F. Uber eine eigenartige rhinogene Granulomatose mit besonderer Beteiligung des Arteriensysems und der Niere. Beitr Pathol Anat Allg Pathol. 1939;36:36–68.
8. Watts R, Carruthers D, Scott D. Epidemiology of systemic vasculitis: changing incidence or definition? Semin Arthritis Rheum. 1995;25:28–34.
9. Cotch M, Hoffmann G, Yerg D, et al. The epidemiology of Wegener's granulomatosis. Estimates of the 5-yr period prevalence, annual mortality and geographic distribution from population – based data sources. Arthritis Rheum. 1996;39:87–92.
10. Stone JK and the WGET Research Group. Baseline data on patients in the Wegener's Granulomatosis Etanercept Trial (WGET): comparisons of the limited and severe disease subsets. Arthritis Rheum. 2003;48:2299–309.
11. Hagen EC, Daha MR, Hermans J, et al. Diagnostic value of standardized assays for anti-neutrophil cytoplasmic antibodies in idiopathic systemic vasculitis. Kidney Int. 1998;53:743–53.
12. Trocme SD, et al. Eosinophil and neutrophil degranulation in ophthalmic lesions of Wegener's granulomatosis. Arch Ophthalmol. 1991;109:1585–9.
13. Coutu RE, et al. Limited form of Wegener's granulomatosis. Eye involvement as a major sign. JAMA. 1975;233:668–71.
14. Messmer EM, Foster CS. Vasculitic peripheral ulcerative keratitis. Surv Ophthalmol. 1999;43: 379–96.
15. Bullen CL, et al. Ocular complications of Wegener's granulomatosis. Ophthalmology. 1983;90:279–90.
16. Robin JB, et al. Ocular involvement in the respiratory vasculitides. Surv Ophthalmol. 1985;30:127–40.
17. Weiter J, Farkas TG. Pseudotumor of the orbit as a presenting sign in Wegener's granulomatosis. Surv Ophthalmol. 1972;17:106–19.
18. Allen JC, France TD. Pseudotumor as the presenting sign of Wegener's granulomatosis in a child. J Pediatr Ophthalmol. 1977;14:158–9.
19. Parelhoff ES, Chavis RM, Friendly DS. Wegener's granulomatosis presenting as orbital pseudotumor in children. J Pediatr Ophthalmol Strabismus. 1985;22:100–4.
20. Coppeto JR, Yarnase H, Monteiro ML. Chronic ophthalmic Wegener's granulomatosis. J Clin Neuroophthalmol. 1985;5:17–25.
21. Perry SR, Rootman J, White VA. The clinical and pathologic constellation of Wegener's granulomatosis of the orbit. Ophthalmology. 1997;104:683–94.
22. Talar-Williams C, Sneller MC, Langford CA, et al. Orbital socket contracture: a complication of inflammatory orbital disease in patients with Wegener's granulomatosis. Br J Ophthalmol. 2005;89:493–7.
23. Haynes BF, et al. The ocular manifestations of Wegener's granulomatosis. Fifteen years experience and review of the literature. Am J Med. 1977;63:131–41.
24. Robinson MR, et al. Tarsal-conjunctival disease associated with Wegener's granulomatosis. Ophthalmology. 2003;1110:1770–80.
25. Tullo AB, et al. Florid xanthelasmata (yellow lids) in orbital Wegener's granulomatosis. Br J Ophthalmol. 1995;79:453–6.
26. Sneller MC. Wegener's granulomatosis. JAMA. 1995;273:1288–91.

27. Leavitt RY, Fauci AS, Block DA, et al. The American College of Rheumatology 1990 criteria for the classification of Wegener's granulomatosis. Arthritis Rheum. 1990;331:1101–7.
28. Walton E. Giant cell granuloma of the respiratory tract (Wegener's granulomatosis). Br Med J. 1958;2:265–70.
29. Hoffman G, Kerr G, Leavitt R, et al. Wegener's granulomatosis: an analysis of 158 patients. Arch Intern Med. 1992;116:488–99.
30. Churg J, Strauss L. Allergic granulomatosis, allergic angiitis and periarteritis nodosa. Am J Pathol. 1951;27:277–301.
31. Lanham JG, Elkon KB, Pusey CD, et al. Systemic vasculitis with asthma and eosinophilia: a clinical approach to the Churg-Strauss syndrome. Medicine (Baltimore). 1984;63:65–81.
32. Sable-Fourtassou R, Cohen P, Mahr A, et al. Antineutrophil cytoplasmic antibodies and the Churg-Strauss syndrome. Ann Intern Med. 2005;43:632–8.
33. Golnik KC. Neuro-ophthalmologic manifestations of systemic disease: rheumatologic/inflammatory. Ophthalmol Clin North Am. 2004;17(3):389–96.
34. Masi AT, Hunder GG, Lie JT, et al. The American College of Rheumatology 1990 criteria for the classification of Churg-Strauss syndrome (allergic granulomatosis and angiitis). Arthritis Rheum. 1990;33:1094–100.
35. Cohen P, Pagnoux C, Mahr A, et al. Churg-Strauss syndrome with poor-prognostic factors: a prospective multicentre trial comparing glucocorticoids and six or twelve cyclophosphamide pulses in 48 patients. Arthritis Rheum. 2007;57:686–93.
36. Flossman O, Berden AE, de Groot K, et al. Long term patient survival in ANCA-associated vasculitis. Ann Rheum Dis. 2011;70:488–4924.
37. Mukhtyar C, Guillevin L, Cid MC, et al. EULAR recommendations for the management of primary small and medium vessel vasculitis. Ann Rheum Dis. 2009;68:310–7.

Orbital Xanthogranulomatous Diseases

7

Zachary D. Pearce and Adam S. Hassan

7.1 Introduction

Xanthogranulomatous diseases of the eyelids and orbit represent a rare group of histiocytic, granulomatous disorders similar in their predominant cell types but diverse in their prognosis – from benign and self-limited to systemically malignant and ultimately fatal. Distinct clinical syndromes involving xanthogranulomatous inflammation have been described, but clinical overlap exists, suggesting that they are part of a continuum. As the name implies, juvenile xanthogranuloma (JXG) affects children. In adults, the four syndromes of xanthogranulomatous inflammation in the eye and adnexa are adult orbital xanthogranuloma (AOX), adult-onset asthma and periocular xanthogranuloma (AAPOX), necrobiotic xanthogranuloma (NXG), and Erdheim-Chester disease (ECD).

7.2 Pathogenesis

Xanthogranulomatous diseases are abnormal proliferations of histiocytes, which are bone marrow-derived stem cells that either develop into dendritic cells or enter the mononuclear

phagocytic system [1, 2]. Dendritic cells become antigen-presenting cells of the skin, known as Langerhans cells. The mononuclear phagocytic system produces phagocytic monocytes, as well as macrophages, both free and fixed tissues [2]. Xanthogranulomatous diseases are abnormal reactive proliferations of non-Langerhans histiocytes, particularly free-tissue macrophages [2]. It is hypothesized that a granulomatous reaction in the skin develops as an immune response to an antigen [3]. Circulating immunoglobulins may form immune complexes that are deposited into periorbital tissues and stimulate the giant cell reaction [3, 4]. No consensus has been made regarding an external stimulus, but limited reports suggest infectious etiologies, such as *Borrelia* and *Cytomegalovirus* may be at play [2, 3]. In addition, JXG patients may show chromosomal instability within circulating immune cells and at the site of inflammation, but no genetic pattern has been identified to date [2, 5].

7.3 Clinical Features

Clinically, xanthogranulomatous diseases present with periocular skin lesions that exist in about 72 % of cases [6]. Typically, these lesions appear as bilateral yellow-orange nodules or plaques and, unlike xanthelasma, tend to be deeper, indurated, and locally invasive and may have a tendency to ulcerate [7]. Infiltration into the lacrimal

Z.D. Pearce, DO (✉) • A.S. Hassan, MD
Department of Ophthalmology, Eye Plastic and Facial Cosmetic Surgery, Grand Rapids, MI, USA
e-mail: pearceza@hotmail.com

H. Demirci (ed.), *Orbital Inflammatory Diseases and Their Differential Diagnosis*,
Essentials in Ophthalmology, DOI 10.1007/978-3-662-46528-8_7,
© Springer-Verlag Berlin Heidelberg 2015

gland may cause globe displacement and aqueous tear deficiency [5]. Orbital masses may present with proptosis, diplopia, restricted ocular motility, and optic neuropathy.

7.4   Diagnostic Evaluation

Diagnostically, xanthogranulomatous diseases are utterly reliant upon histopathology and immunohistochemistry. The microscopic hallmark is dense infiltrates of foamy histiocytes (xanthoma cells), Touton (and sometimes foreign body) giant cells, plasma cells, and lymphocytes with variable fibrosis [5, 6, 8, 9]. Oil Red O staining confirms the lipid content of the xanthoma cells on frozen specimens [5]. Touton giant cells characteristically have an eosinophilic core, surrounded by a ring of numerous nuclei, with a peripheral rim of translucent, foamy cytoplasm near the cell membrane [10]. Necrosis is most marked in NXG but may be seen in other syndromes [6]. As a rule, immunohistochemistry reveals cells that are CD68 and factor XIIIa positive [2, 5, 6]. Langerhans cell histiocytoses are excluded by the absence of staining for CD1a and S-100 [5, 8, 11]. Absence of Birbeck granules on electron microscopy also confirms the diagnosis by excluding a Langerhans cell lineage [2, 11]. Although few case reports of AOX and ECD have been S-100 positive and shown the presence of Birbeck granules in ECD, most cases display a similar pattern [5, 12]. Table 7.1 summarizes the differentiation of xanthogranulomatous diseases from Langerhans cell histiocytoses.

In two series, neuroimaging revealed poorly defined, infiltrative soft tissue masses with increased fat (66 %), extraocular muscle enlargement (suggesting infiltration) (100 %), optic nerve encasement (38 %), and lacrimal gland enlargement (56–63 %) [2, 5, 7]. Orbital lesions typically mold to the globe and do not usually cause destruction of the bony walls of the orbit [2, 7]. In JXG, radiographic evidence of optic nerve encasement, bony destruction, and intracranial extension has been described [7].

Table 7.1 Differentiating xanthogranulomatous diseases from Langerhans cell histiocytoses

Xanthogranulomatous diseases	Langerhans cell histiocytoses
Positive for	Positive for
CD68	CD1a
Factor XIIIa	S-100
Negative for	Birbeck granules on electron microscopy
CD1a	Negative for
S-100	CD68
Birbeck granules on electron microscopy	Factor XIIIa

7.5   Juvenile Xanthogranuloma (JXG)

Juvenile xanthogranuloma classically presents as multiple yellow-red papules on the face, neck, axillae, and extensor surfaces of the extremities, which range in size from 0.5 cm to several centimeters in diameter [5, 9, 13, 14]. The average age of onset is 2 years, with no sex predilection. Cutaneous manifestations are usually self-limited and resolve spontaneously within 2 years. Extracutaneous involvement has been described, including the heart, lungs, liver, testes, and hematopoietic system [5, 9]. The eye, however, is the most common site to be affected after the skin. The most common ocular manifestation of JXG is iris infiltration leading to spontaneous hyphema and treatment-resistant secondary glaucoma [5, 13]. Also described is involvement of the eyelid, conjunctiva, cornea, episclera, uveal tract, optic nerve, and orbit [9]. Orbital involvement is extremely rare, with 80 % of orbital JXG lacking the typical skin findings [10, 13].

Systemic evaluation for potential malignancies should be considered because other organ systems may be affected [14]. Specifically in the setting of neurofibromatosis type 1 (NF-1), JXG has been associated with an increased rate of myelomonocytic leukemia [14]. Biopsy of any orbital mass is necessary to rule out malignancy, such as rhabdomyosarcoma, and secure a diagnosis.

Observation is usually recommended because most lesions resolve spontaneously [5, 9, 14, 15].

Topical, oral, and intralesional corticosteroids have been used with success in the setting of an associated systemic disease or if an amblyogenic mass is present [9, 13, 14]. Surgical excision has been successful in solitary masses with only a rare risk of recurrence [14]. External radiotherapy has also been used sparingly for refractory cases, but the risk of secondary head and neck malignancies limits its use [13, 14].

7.6 Adult Orbital Xanthogranuloma (AOX)

An isolated xanthogranulomatous lesion without significant systemic involvement is classified as adult orbital xanthogranuloma. This is the least common of these syndromes and is really a diagnosis of exclusion. The diffuse, yellow-orange, elevated, indurated eyelid plaque is virtually diagnostic of AOX and tends to affect the eyelids and anterior orbital tissues, producing mild proptosis [6, 10, 16]. It is a disease of middle-aged to elderly adults without sex predilection and often involves both sides. Biopsy is necessary to rule out necrosis. Systemic evaluation is necessary to rule out immunologic disease, asthma, Erdheim-Chester disease, and hyperlipidemia. It is often self-limited and does not require aggressive treatment [5]. Intralesional corticosteroid injection has been successfully used in controlling adult-onset xanthogranuloma [16, 17].

Figure 7.1 is an external photograph of a patient with biopsy-proven adult orbital xanthogranulomatosis.

7.7 Adult-Onset Asthma and Periocular Xanthogranuloma (AAPOX)

Adult-onset asthma and periocular xanthogranuloma is a rare condition, first reported by Jakobiec in 1993 [18]. The range of reported cases is 22–74 years of age, with a 2:1 male to female preponderance [5]. Typically, bilateral, elevated, non-ulcerated, yellow-orange xanthomatous

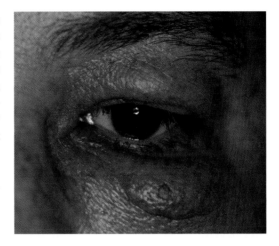

Fig. 7.1 External photograph of a patient with biopsy-proven adult orbital xanthogranulomatosis. Note the erythematous, indurated, periorbital mass with focal ulceration

lesions affect the eyelids and may extend into the anterior orbital fat, as well as infiltrate the extraocular muscles and lacrimal gland [5, 18]. The yellow skin plaques may be preceded by diffuse periorbital swelling by as much as 5 years [10]. Biopsy shows the classic xanthogranulomatous infiltrate and Touton giant cells but lacks necrosis [18]. It often contains germinal centers and scattered eosinophils.

As the name implies, systemic association can include adult-onset asthma that may present within a few months to a few years of the eyelid lesions [5, 19]. Asthma is just one of the many types of immune dysfunction frequently seen in adult patients with orbital xanthogranulomatous diseases. Others include autoimmune thyrotoxicosis, paraproteinemia, lymphadenopathy, and other lymphoproliferative disorders (multiple myeloma, chronic lymphocytic leukemia, benign lymphoproliferation, non-Hodgkin's lymphoma, Hodgkin's lymphoma, and Burkitt lymphoma) [5, 6]. In fact, Sivak et al. found evidence of immune dysfunction in all pooled cases of AAPOX and NXG [6]. Therefore, thorough evaluation and close follow-up by a hematologist/oncologist is recommended [5, 18].

Treatments for AAPOX have been broad, with varying results. Systemic corticosteroids may cause temporary improvement, but their long-term efficacy is questionable [5]. Cytotoxic and chemotherapy agents have been tried in limited series with significant improvement in some but were limited by side effects [5, 20]. Surgical debulking helps but may cause significant inflammatory reaction and scarring, as well as recurrence after 6–12 months [5, 18]. In another series by Elner et al., multiple (1–22) intralesional corticosteroid injections either stabilized or improved all six patients with AOX and NXG [16]. It might be possible to extrapolate this data to AAPOX patients, with little adverse risk. Despite no consensus to the best treatment, overall prognosis is still good [6].

7.8 Necrobiotic Xanthogranuloma (NXG)

Necrobiotic xanthogranuloma was initially described in 1980 by Kossard and in 1984 by Robertson and Winkelmann [21, 22, 23]. NXG manifests in 20–95-year-olds, but typically the sixth decade, with no sex predilection [5, 23]. Skin lesions are described as yellow, indurated nodules or plaques that are slowly progressive and relentlessly destructive [4, 19]. Ulceration is a predominant feature and is present in 42 % of cases [3, 4, 10, 23]. Skin lesions on the trunk and extremities are the initial presenting sign in 65 % of cases [4]. It affects the ocular adnexa, periorbital skin, trunk, and flexure surfaces of the extremities [4]. Cutaneous involvement is present in nearly all cases, with a clear predilection for periorbital tissues, but the classic periorbital lesions may be absent in 15 % of cases [4, 23]. Ocular manifestations are present in about 81 % of NXG and are usually limited to the eyelids and anterior orbit but may include cellulitis, proptosis, episcleritis, keratitis, uveitis, and dacryoadenitis [4, 6, 16, 19]. Periorbital skin changes may lead to exposure keratopathy, corneal ulceration, and, ultimately, perforation as in reports by Reddy and Oestreicher [4, 23]. Histologically, typical Touton and foreign body giant cells are present, but NXG is distinct from the other xanthogranulomatoses by the presence of necrosis and cholesterol clefts [4, 19]. NXG shows

necrobiosis of collagen surrounded by palisading epithelioid histiocytes.

There is a clear association with paraproteinemias, which exists in 80–90 % of NXG cases [4, 19, 23]. IgG monoclonal gammopathy is the most common disorder, specifically kappa light chain in 65 % [3, 10]. Approximately 50 % of these paraproteinemias and blood disorders progress to hematologic malignancies, such as multiple myeloma, non-Hodgkin's lymphoma, and chronic lymphocytic leukemia [3, 4, 10, 17, 19]. An elevated erythrocyte sedimentation rate, low serum complement, and occasional mild hyperlipidemia are accompanying hematologic abnormalities [10]. Eleven percent of NXG patients also had evidence of internal organ disease (heart, lung, kidney, liver, intestine, spleen, ovary, and pharynx) [3].

Many treatment modalities have been employed with varying degrees of success, and unfortunately, the lifelong risk of hematologic malignancies does not seem to be affected by treatments [3]. Systemic corticosteroids may help temporarily [5]. As noted previously, in a small series of AOX and NXG patients, intralesional corticosteroid injections were effective at stabilizing or improving all cases after multiple injections [16]. Ugurlu et al. noted improvement in 22 % of NXG patients treated with local corticosteroid injection, but the number of injections was not specified [24]. Adjunctive chemotherapy with chlorambucil, methotrexate, azathioprine, melphalan, and interferon has shown some benefit [4, 5]. Radiation has been used successfully in some small case series, but the reports are equivocal [5]. In a retrospective review of four cases (2 ECD, 1 NXG, 1 AOX) by Ebrahimi et al., none of the patients improved with radiotherapy, with 3 of 4 patients experiencing an acute exacerbation of their disease [25]. Surgical excision is generally not recommended because of the mechanical trauma and resultant inflammation that occurs. Lesion recurrences have occurred in 42 % of cases 6–12 months after excision [4, 24]. The recurrences were often larger than the original lesions. Necrobiotic xanthogranulomatous reaction has also been noted to occur at surgical sites that were previously unaffected, such as after an appendectomy and saphenous vein graft [4, 26]. NXG remains a challenging entity to treat due to its systemic involvement and persistent course.

7.9 Erdheim-Chester Disease (ECD)

Of the adult xanthogranulomatous conditions, Erdheim-Chester disease is the most worrisome. While the ocular presentations of these diseases are quite similar, ECD has systemic associations that make the condition fatal. First described in 1930, ECD is a systemic xanthogranulomatous process that is associated with radiographic alterations in the bone [27]. It affects adults with a mean age of 54, and like AAPOX, men are affected twice as often as women [5, 12]. As in the other xanthogranulomatoses, large, markedly xanthomatous histiocytes, Touton giant cells, lymphocytes, plasma cells, and variable degree of fibrosis are found in the lesion. A pattern of CD68+, factor XIIIa+, Cd1a-, and S-100- predominates immunohistochemistry [19, 27]. Birbeck granules are not present on electron microscopy [19].

Although rare, when ECD affects the orbit, it is usually bilateral, diffuse, and intraconal and prefers the posterior portion of the orbit [8, 16, 28]. The orbital masses may precede eyelid xanthelasmic lesions by several years [11]. The orbital masses may cause compression of the optic nerve with subsequent optic disc edema, visual field constriction, and progressive vision loss [8, 11]. Two patterns of ocular involvement of ECD have been suggested by Hoffmann. The first has mild visual impairment, but the second has progressive loss of vision despite treatment [8].

Systemic involvement of ECD includes a nearly pathognomonic symmetrical pattern of histiocytic infiltration of long tubular bones, as seen on plain x-rays and technetium-99m bone scan [19]. Bony involvement typically spares the axial skeleton and shows sclerosis of the metaphysis and diaphysis of long tubular bones [11, 12]. This is vital to the diagnosis and present in 100 % of cases of ECD [27]. The infiltrative nature of this systemic disease can be widespread, and

death is usually due to vital organ compromise. Classic findings include pericardial or pleural effusion, retroperitoneal involvement (in approximately 50 %), perinephric or mediastinal infiltrates, diabetes insipidus (due to pituitary infiltration), brain/dural masses, and hepatosplenomegaly [6, 16, 27]. In a series by Sivak, all 22 cases of ECD had internal organ disease [6]. Biopsy of any systemic lesion will show the same histiocytic infiltrate as the orbital mass [2].

Treatment recommendations include observation, systemic steroids, radiotherapy, chemotherapy (methotrexate, cyclophosphamide, doxorubicin, vincristine), and interferon-α [5, 11]. In the setting of progressive visual loss, orbital decompression may be indicated [11]. ECD is often aggressive despite treatment and the prognosis is related to the extent of visceral involvement. Most patients die within the first year from congestive heart failure, cardiomyopathy, lung fibrosis, or renal insufficiency [5, 11].

7.10 Summary

Orbital xanthogranulomatous diseases are a spectrum of disorders that can provide clues to serious systemic illnesses. Clinical suspicion with, or without, the presence of indurated, yellow eyelid plaques or orbital masses should prompt biopsy. Histologically, the typical foamy histiocytic infiltration with giant cells and fibrosis suggest this group of conditions. Immunohistochemistry revealing CD68 positive, factor XIIIa positive, CD1a negative, and S-100 negative will confirm the diagnosis. Hematologic workup should be initiated promptly and followed long term, especially in the setting of children with NF-1, necrosis on histology, ulceration of the skin lesions, or symmetric involvement of the long tubular bones. Long bone involvement on x-ray or technetium-99m bone scan should also prompt a systemic evaluation for vital organ infiltration. This should include an echocardiogram and imaging of the chest and abdomen. Treatment recommendations include observation, intralesional corticosteroids, systemic corticosteroids, chemotherapy agents, and radiotherapy. Some sources imply that surgical excision may worsen local xanthogranu-lomatous disease and should be used cautiously, especially in adult cases. Despite aggressive treatments, clinical response may vary, and the treatment regimen should be dictated by the clini-cal course and associated systemic involvement. Unquestionably, early recognition of these enti-ties provides the best potential prognosis for these potentially devastating disorders.

Compliance with Ethical Standards Zachary D. Pearce and Adam S. Hassan declare that they have no conflict of interest. No human studies were carried out by the authors for this article. No animal studies were carried out by the authors for this article.

References

1. Cruz AA, de Alencar VM, Falcão MF, Elias Jr J, Chahud F. Association between Erdheim-Chester dis-ease, Hashimoto thyroiditis, and familial thrombocyto-penia. Ophthal Plast Reconstr Surg. 2006;22(1):60–2.
2. Karcioglu ZA, Sharara N, Boles TL, Nasr AM. Orbital xanthogranuloma: clinical and morphologic features in eight patients. Ophthal Plast Reconstr Surg. 2003; 19(5):372–81.
3. Hawryluk EB, Izikson L, English 3rd JC. Non-infectious granulomatous diseases of the skin and their associated systemic diseases: an evidence-based update to important clinical questions. Am J Clin Dermatol. 2010;11(3):171–81.
4. Oestreicher J, Dookeran R, Nijhawan N, Kolin A. Necrobiotic xanthogranuloma with predominant periorbital involvement. Ophthal Plast Reconstr Surg. 2010;26(6):473–5.
5. Guo J, Wang J. Adult orbital xanthogranulomatous disease: review of the literature. Arch Pathol Lab Med. 2009;133(12):1994–7.
6. Sivak-Callcott JA, Rootman J, Rasmussen SL, Nugent RA, White VA, Paridaens D, Currie Z, Rose G, Clark B, McNab AA, Buffam FV, Neigel JM, Kazim M. Adult xanthogranulomatous disease of the orbit and ocular adnexa: new immunohistochemical findings and clini-cal review. Br J Ophthalmol. 2006;90(5):602–8.
7. Miszkiel KA, Sohaib SA, Rose GE, Cree IA, Moseley IF. Radiological and clinicopathological features of orbital xanthogranuloma. Br J Ophthalmol. 2000; 84(3):251–8.
8. Hoffmann EM, Müller-Forell W, Pitz S, Radner H. Erdheim-Chester disease: a case report. Graefes Arch Clin Exp Ophthalmol. 2004;242(9):803–7.
9. Mruthyunjaya P, Meyer DR. Juvenile xanthogranu-loma of the lacrimal sac fossa. Am J Ophthalmol. 1997;123(3):400–2.
10. Rose GE, Patel BC, Garner A, Wright JE. Orbital xan-thogranuloma in adults. Br J Ophthalmol. 1991; 75(11):680–4.
11. Valmaggia C, Neuweiler J, Fretz C, Gottlob I. A case of Erdheim-Chester disease with orbital involvement. Arch Ophthalmol. 1997;115(11):1467–8.
12. Kenn W, Staebler A, Zachoval R, et al. Erdheim-Chester disease: a case report and literature overview. Eur Radiol. 1999;9:153–8.
13. Shields CL, Shields JA, Buchanon HW. Solitary orbital involvement with juvenile xanthogranuloma. Arch Ophthalmol. 1990;108(11):1587–9.
14. Kuruvilla R, Escaravage Jr GK, Finn AJ, Dutton JJ. Infiltrative subcutaneous juvenile xanthogranu-loma of the eyelid in a neonate. Ophthal Plast Reconstr Surg. 2009;25(4):330–2.
15. Johnson TE, Alabiad C, Wei L, Davis JA. Extensive juvenile xanthogranuloma involving the orbit, sinuses, brain, and subtemporal fossa in a newborn. Ophthal Plast Reconstr Surg. 2010;26(2):133–4.
16. Elner VM, Mintz R, Demirci H, Hassan AS. Local cor-ticosteroid treatment of eyelid and orbital xanthogranu-loma. Trans Am Ophthalmol Soc. 2005;103:69–73.
17. Elner VM, Mintz R, Demirci H, Hassan AS. Local corticosteroid treatment of eyelid and orbital xantho-granuloma. Ophthal Plast Reconstr Surg. 2006;22(1): 36–40.
18. Tokuhara KG, Agarwal MR, Rao NA. Adult-onset asthma and severe periocular xanthogranuloma: a case report. Ophthal Plast Reconstr Surg. 2011;27(3): e63–4.
19. Hammond MD, Niemi EW, Ward TP, Eiseman AS. Adult orbital xanthogranuloma with associated adult-onset asthma. Ophthal Plast Reconstr Surg. 2004;20(4):329–32.
20. Hayden A, Wilson DJ, Rosenbaum JT. Management of orbital xanthogranuloma with methotrexate. Br J Ophthalmol. 2007;91(4):434–6.
21. Kossard S, Winkelmann RK. Necrobiotic xantho-granuloma with proteinemia. J Am Acad Dermatol. 1980;3(3):257–70.
22. Robertson DM, Winkelmann RK. Ophthalmic fea-tures of necrobiotic xanthogranuloma with parapro-teinemia. Am J Ophthalmol. 1984;97(2):173–83.
23. Reddy VC, Salomão DR, Garrity JA, Baratz KH, Patel SV. Periorbital and ocular necrobiotic xantho-granuloma leading to perforation. Arch Ophthalmol. 2010;128(11):1493–4.
24. Ugurlu S, Bartley GB, Gibson LE. Necrobiotic xan-thogranuloma: long-term outcome of ocular and sys-temic involvement. Am J Ophthalmol. 2000;129: 651–7.
25. Ebrahimi KB, Miller NR, Sassani JW, Iliff NT, Green WR. Failure of radiation therapy in orbital xantho-granuloma. Ophthal Plast Reconstr Surg. 2010;26(4): 259–64.
26. Rayner SA, Duncombe AS, Keefe M, Theaker J, Manners RM. Necrobiotic xanthogranuloma occur-ring in an eyelid scar. Orbit. 2008;27(3):191–4.
27. de Palma P, Ravalli L, Grisanti F, Rossi A, Marzola A, Nielsen I. Bilateral orbital involvement in Erdheim-Chester disease. Orbit. 1998;17(2):97–105.
28. Malhotra R, Porter RG, Selva D. Adult orbital xanthogranuloma with periosteal infiltration. Br J Ophthalmol. 2003;87(1):120–1.

Langerhans Cell Histiocytosis

8

Zachary D. Pearce, Hakan Demirci,
and Adam S. Hassan

8.1   Introduction

Langerhans cell histiocytosis (LCH) represents a
spectrum of disorders with consistent histopathologic characteristics, but marked phenotypic and
prognostic variability. Although much knowledge has been gained regarding this disease process, clinical patterns continue to inspire debate
among physicians. A thorough understanding of
the historical perspectives of the disease, current
classification systems, as well as the perspectives
among different medical specialties is important
in caring for these patients.

8.2   Historical Perspective

Langerhans cells were originally described by
Paul Langerhans, while a medical student, who
mistakenly thought these cells of the skin were
nerve cells due to their dendritic configuration.

Z.D. Pearce, DO (✉) • A.S. Hassan, MD
Department of Ophthalmology,
Eye Plastic and Facial Cosmetic Surgery,
Grand Rapids, MI, USA
e-mail: pearceza@hotmail.com

H. Demirci, MD
Department of Ophthalmology and Visual Sciences,
W.K. Kellogg Eye Center, University of Michigan,
Ann Arbor, MI, USA
e-mail: hdemirci@umich.edu

These cells are now known to originate from a
myeloid progenitor precursor in the bone marrow
and, by cytokine stimulation, mature to become
an antigen-presenting cell of the epidermis,
mucous membranes, lymph nodes, and spleen [1].
Constituting an early barrier to pathogens, they
are an important part of the immune system.

Normally in the bone marrow, Langerhans
cells are formed from pluripotent precursors and,
by means of cytokine influence such as
granulocyte-macrophage colony-stimulating factor (GM-CSF), tumor necrosis factor alpha
(TNF-α), and interleukin-1 (IL-1), may become
activated to process antigens and present to T
lymphocytes [1]. It is thought that several different events may trigger an alteration of cytokine
production, such as localized trauma, infection,
or some pathologic genetic abnormality. This
"cytokine storm" allows for maturational arrest
and unregulated proliferation of pathologic
Langerhans cells, forming a soft tissue mass with
adjacent bony destruction. It is usually a monoclonal proliferation of histiocytes with granuloma formation and an infiltrate of eosinophilic
and neutrophilic inflammatory cells [1, 2].
Immunohistochemistry of Langerhans cells is
historically positive for CD1a, S100, and, more
recently, langerin (CD207) [1, 3]. Transmission
electron microscopy shows Birbeck granules,
which are racquet-shaped intracytoplasmic
organelles and are pathognomonic, but not necessary for diagnosis [1]. Older lesions may show

varying degrees of necrosis, fibrosis, or even mitotic figures, which have no correlation with disease severity [1].

Adjacent to the soft tissue mass in LCH, bony destruction is often present and thought to be related to interleukin-1 (IL-1) and prostaglandin E2 (PGE2), as part of the "cytokine storm" [4]. IL-1 inhibits bone formation by disrupting collagen formation and osteoclast activity, whereas PGE2 induces bone resorption [3, 4]. These two cytokines represent potential targeted therapies, such as corticosteroids, which inhibit IL-1 bone resorption and PGE2 production [4]. TNF-α may also contribute to inflammatory bone destruction and nonspecific systemic complications [3].

8.3   Etiologies

The pathogenesis of LCH is related to an aberrant immune system, but the exact etiology is often a topic of debate. Possible causes include infections (Epstein-Barr virus, cytomegalovirus, human herpes virus 6), genetic disorders (BRAF mutation), malignancies (leukemia, Hodgkin's disease, medulloblastoma, retinoblastoma, medullary astrocytoma, glioma), and seasonal/environmental influences such as minor trauma [1]. In a case series by Herwig et al., four of five cases of orbital LCH had a preceding history of local trauma [1]. In another case series, the BRAF gene mutation was found in more than half of their LCH patients [3]. Despite the many theories, however, no single factor has been uniformly implicated to date.

The variable biologic behavior sparks debate over LCH being an inflammatory or neoplastic process. The possibility of a traumatic etiology and spontaneous resolution in milder forms suggest an inflammatory course. The granulomatous histologic pattern is also consistent with inflammation. Most cases, however, show a monoclonal proliferation which is suggestive of a malignant process. Patients with BRAF mutation are more likely to have reactivation of their disease, suggesting a genetic predisposition [3]. The inconsistency of trigger events, presence of genetic defects, and potentially unrelenting and grave clinical course may also suggest neoplasia.

8.4   Epidemiology

LCH is a rare disease with an estimated incidence of up to four to five cases per million per year in children [4–6]. The involved age groups vary by clinical presentation. Multisystem LCH usually occurs before 3 years of age, and unifocal disease is more common in later childhood [7]. Ocular adnexal LCH often presents between 4 and 8 years old [8]. Less commonly, LCH may present in adulthood, with a mean age of 35 years [1]. Males are more frequently affected than females, reaching ratios of 2:1 in some studies [9]. Females, however, may have more severe organ involvement [1]. Caucasians are more commonly affected [1]. Single-system disease represents approximately 70 % of cases [10]. It is usually sporadic, but genetic influence may exist, as 1 % of LCH patients have an affected relative [3].

8.5   Classification

Currently, LCH is divided according to the guidelines of the Histiocytosis Society, as shown in Table 8.1. The two major categories are single system (SS) or multisystem (MS). SS LCH is further subdivided into single site (unifocal bone, skin, or lymph node) or multiple sites (multifocal bone or multiple lymph nodes). MS LCH is defined as involvement of two or more organs at diagnosis, with or without organ dysfunction. MS LCH may be further subdivided into low- and high-risk groups, by risk organ involvement (risk organ positive and risk organ negative). High-risk organ sites include liver, lungs, spleen, and widespread bone marrow due to their higher associated mortality (10–50 %), despite intensive treatment [1, 10, 11]. Survival

Table 8.1 Classification scheme of Langerhans cell histiocytosis

Single system (SS)	Multisystem (MS)
Unifocal (bone, skin, lymph node)	Low risk
Multifocal (bone or lymph nodes)	High-risk organ involvement (liver, spleen, lung, hematopoietic)

of SS or MS disease without risk organ involvement approaches 100 % [10].

Children with SS LCH represent about 70 % of cases and most commonly affect bone (unifocal or multifocal) [10]. The most common presenting clinical manifestations are a soft tissue mass with adjacent bone involvement and pain, skin rash, fever, and lymphadenopathy [10].

8.5.1 Bone

Overall, 80 % of LCH cases involve the bone [10]. In children, the skull is most commonly affected, followed by the spine, extremities, pelvis, and ribs [10]. In adults, the jaw is most often affected [10]. When the bone is solely involved, the clinical course is often benign, and spontaneous resolution may occur [10].

8.5.2 Skin

Dermatologic involvement is present in about half of cases, frequently in infants [10]. Clinical description is variable and includes erythema, papules, nodules, petechiae, vesicles, crusted plaques, and seborrhea-like eruptions [10]. Systemic evaluation is mandatory with cutaneous involvement because MS LCH disease is the norm, and death may occur [10].

8.5.3 Lungs

Pulmonary involvement is usually MS LCH in children, but SS LCH in adults [10]. It is important to note that adult pulmonary LCH has been associated with smoking and may regress with smoking cessation [10]. However, adult pulmonary LCH has also been reported to have a mortality of up to 25 % [10].

8.5.4 Hematopoietic

When diffuse bone marrow involvement is present, life-threatening anemia and thrombocytopenia may result [10].

8.5.5 Hypothalamic-Pituitary Dysfunction

Twenty-five percent of all LCH and 50 % of multisystem LCH may have dysfunction or infiltration of the pituitary gland or hypothalamus [10]. Diabetes insipidus (DI) may occur at any time of the disease course and is more frequently associated with craniofacial bone lesions, ear, eye, and/or oral lesions [10]. Therefore, these systems are referred to as "CNS risk lesions" [10]. Appropriate chemotherapy may prevent DI, but rarely cures it. Approximately 50 % of patients with DI develop other pituitary hormone abnormalities [10]. Other central nervous system (CNS) lesions include bilateral symmetric cerebellar and basal ganglia lesions that result in progressive ataxia, tremor, dysarthria, dysphasia, hyperreflexia, and permanent disability [10]. This may occur in approximately half of patients with DI and/or other CNS risk lesions [10].

8.5.6 Ocular and Orbital Manifestations

Solitary orbital lesions are by far the most common ocular manifestation and carry a favorable prognosis [1]. A soft tissue mass with an associated osteolytic bony lesion with sclerotic margin is often seen. The frontal bone is most commonly affected, followed by the lateral and medial orbital walls [2]. The mean age of onset is 4 years, with a range of 18 months to 30 years [2]. Presenting signs and symptoms include ptosis, proptosis, periorbital erythema, edema, amblyopia, or diplopia/strabismus [1]. Lesions involving the eyelid, conjunctiva, caruncle, choroid, orbital apex, optic chiasm, and cavernous sinus have been described [1]. Orbital LCH represents less than 1 % of all orbital tumors and inflammatory lesions [8]. Although LCH of the orbit is most commonly isolated (single system), it may be part of multisystem (MS) disease, so full systemic workup is imperative.

The implications of orbital lesions, however, are a topic of debate. In previous multicenter trials by the Histiocyte Society, patients with diabetes insipidus were twice as likely to have orbital lesions, leading the authors to conclude that the orbital involvement is a risk factor for DI [12, 13]. However, all of the cases developing DI had multisystem LCH along with their orbital lesions, and none had unifocal LCH of the orbit. Harris rebutted the conclusion that orbital involvement was a risk factor for DI, stating that he was not aware of any reported case of unifocal orbital LCH that later developed DI or CNS disease [4]. A recent multivariate meta-analysis by the Histiocyte Society appears to support Harris' concept by showing that only auditory system and multisystem diseases are significant risk factors for DI and CNS disease, particularly the pituitary-hypothalamic region [14, 15].

8.6 Diagnosis/Workup

Because LCH may be part of a multisystem disorder, a complete history and physical examination is necessary. Localized imaging by CT or MRI is required, as well as full body imaging such as skull x-ray, complete bone survey/bone scan/PET scan, chest x-ray, and abdomen/pelvis imaging. Systemic workup includes complete blood cell count with differential, erythrocyte sedimentation rate, electrolytes, coagulation profile, liver function testing, urinalysis with osmolarity, water deprivation test, and bone marrow biopsy [1].

Recurrence or progression usually occurs in the first 12–18 months, but later complications have been reported. At least 5 years of follow-up has been recommended [1].

8.7 Treatments

Because the clinical course differs widely in LCH, treatment recommendations may vary from observation to systemic chemotherapy. Isolated (single-system) LCH of the orbit is usually responsive to local treatment, such as curettage,

with or without intralesional corticosteroid injection [4]. Extensive resections are usually not necessary because most of the bone lesions heal spontaneously, even if residual tumor is left after partial surgical debridement [5]. It is proposed that interventions, such as biopsy and partial curettage, may sufficiently alter the pathologic cascade and "reset" the immune system to allow for spontaneous resolution. Any recurrence or sign of systemic disease requires 6–12 months of systemic chemotherapy with vinblastine and corticosteroids [10].

Currently, systemic chemotherapy is recommended for all MS LCH as well as SS LCH with the following features: CNS risk lesions, multifocal bone, and "special sites," such as the odontoid peg or vertebral column with intraspinal extension [16]. Systemic chemotherapy is initiated for 6–12 months, with systemic cytotoxic agents, such as vinblastine, as well as corticosteroids [10]. High-risk organ involvement necessitates more aggressive treatment due to the high mortality. However, as stated previously, it has been debated that an isolated orbital lesion is not actually at increased risk to the central nervous system.

Conclusion

To the ophthalmologist, LCH most frequently represents a solitary bony mass that behaves like an inflammatory lesion and responds very well to surgical curettage and local corticosteroids. The oncologist, however, encounters a potentially fatal systemic malignancy that can be unrelenting despite aggressive treatment. This paradox has long since accompanied the clinical entities now known as Langerhans cell histiocytosis. Understanding the spectrum of the disease and classification schemes, as well as maintaining collaboration between medical specialties, is of the upmost importance in caring for these patients.

Compliance with Ethical Standards Zachary D. Pearce, Adam S. Hassan, and Hakan Demirci declare that they have no conflict of interest. No human studies were carried out by the authors for this article. No animal studies were carried out by the authors for this article.

References

1. Herwig MC, Wojno T, Zhang Q, Grossniklaus HE. Langerhans cell histiocytosis of the orbit: five clinico-pathologic cases and review of the literature. Surv Ophthalmol. 2013;58:330–40.
2. Giovannetti F, Giona F, Ungari C, et al. Langerhans cell histiocytosis with orbital involvement: our experience. J Oral Maxillofac Surg. 2009;67:212–6.
3. Margo CE, Goldman DR. Langerhans cell histiocytosis. Surv Ophthalmol. 2008;53:332–58.
4. Harris GJ. Langerhans cell histiocytosis of the orbit: a need for interdisciplinary dialogue. Am J Ophthalmol. 2006;141:374–8.
5. Harris GJ, Woo KI. Is unifocal Langerhans-cell histiocytosis of the orbit a "CNS-Risk" lesion? Pediatr Blood Cancer. 2004;43(3):298–9, author reply 300–1.
6. Stalemark H, Laurencikas E, Karis J, et al. Incidence of Langerhans cell histiocytosis in children: a population-based study. Pediatr Blood Cancer. 2008;51(1): 76–81.
7. Maccheron LJ, McNab AA, Elder J, et al. Ocular adnexal Langerhans cell histiocytosis clinical features and management. Orbit. 2006;25(3):169–77.
8. Cheung N, Selva D, McNab AA. Orbital Langerhans cell histiocytosis in adults. Ophthalmology. 2007;114: 1569–73.
9. Cochrane LA, Prince M, Clarke K. Langerhans' cell histiocytosis in the paediatric population: presentation and treatment of head and neck manifestations. J Otolaryngol. 2003;32(1):33–7.
10. Morimoto A, Oh Y, Shioda Y, et al. Recent advances in Langerhans cell histiocytosis. Pediatr Int. 2014; 56:451–61.
11. Broadbent V, Gadner H. Current therapy for Langerhans cell histiocytosis. Hematol Oncol Clin North Am. 1998;12(2):327–38.
12. Grois N, Flucher-Wolfram B, Heitger A, et al. Diabetes insipidus in Langerhans cell histiocytosis: results from the DAL-HX 83 study. Med Pediatr Oncol. 1995;24(4):248–56.
13. Haupt R, Nanduri V, Calevo MG, et al. Permanent consequences in Langerhans cell histiocytosis patients: a pilot study from the Histiocyte Society-Late Effects Study Group. Pediatr Blood Cancer. 2004;42(5):438–44.
14. Grois N, Potschger U, Prosch H, et al. Risk factors for diabetes insipidus in langerhans cell histiocytosis. Pediatr Blood Cancer. 2006;46(2):228–33.
15. Grois N, Prayer D, Prosch H, et al. Course and clinical impact of magnetic resonance imaging findings in diabetes insipidus associated with Langerhans cell histiocytosis. Pediatr Blood Cancer. 2004;43(1):59–65.
16. Minov M, Grois N, McClain K, et al. Histiocyte society evaluation and treatment guidelines. http://www.histiocytesociety.org/document.doc?id=290. Apr 2009.

Thyroid Eye Disease: A Comprehensive Review

9

Shannon S. Joseph and Raymond S. Douglas

Core Messages

- Thyroid eye disease (TED) is an auto-immune process closely associated with Graves' disease.
- Orbital fibroblasts are the principal effector cells responsible for orbital soft tissue enlargement in TED through hyaluronan synthesis, cytokine production, and fibroblast differentiation.
- The thyrotropin receptor and insulin-like growth factor-1 receptor are autoantigens that appear to play a central role in the pathogenesis of TED.
- The most common clinical findings of TED include eyelid malposition, exophthalmos, and restrictive strabismus.
- Clinical history and exam form the basis of diagnosis for TED, but abnormalities in thyroid function and immunological tests support the diagnosis.
- Orbital computed tomography is the imaging modality of choice for TED.
- Smoking is the most important modifiable risk factor for TED.

- Euthyroidism should be rapidly achieved and maintained in all patients with TED.
- Conservative measures are the mainstay of treatment for mild TED.
- The current first line of therapy for active moderate-to-severe and sight-threatening TED is intravenous (IV) glucocorticoids.
- Orbital radiotherapy can be used as an adjunctive treatment for select patients with active TED.
- The efficacy of novel disease-modifying agents such as rituximab is under investigation.
- If sight-threatening TED is refractory to IV glucocorticoids, then urgent surgical management is indicated.
- To treat compressive optic neuropathy, surgical decompression needs to focus on the posteromedial orbit, relieving compression at the orbital apex.
- Orbital decompression surgery to reduce exophthalmos can involve orbital fat resection and removal of the lateral wall, medial wall, and, rarely, orbital floor.
- TED must be stable and nonprogressive for at least 6 months prior to surgical rehabilitation.
- TED rehabilitative surgery should be performed in the following sequence: orbital decompression, extraocular muscle surgery, and eyelid surgery.

S.S. Joseph, MD, MSc • R.S. Douglas, MD, PhD (✉)
Department of Ophthalmology,
University of Michigan,
1000 Wall Street, Ann Arbor, MI 48105, USA
e-mail: sjshan@med.umich.edu; raydougl@med.umich.edu

H. Demirci (ed.), *Orbital Inflammatory Diseases and Their Differential Diagnosis*,
Essentials in Ophthalmology, DOI 10.1007/978-3-662-46528-8_9,
© Springer-Verlag Berlin Heidelberg 2015

9.1   Epidemiology

Thyroid eye disease (TED) is an autoimmune phenomenon that can lead to permanent vision loss. Nearly 90 % of cases occur within 18 months of the onset of hyperthyroidism due to Graves' disease (GD) [1–3]. The remaining 10 % are associated with euthyroidism or hypothyroidism [4]. The calculated prevalence of TED in the United States is 0.25 % [2]. However, its prevalence among individuals with GD is much higher, at 20–50 % [2, 5]. Indeed, up to 70 % of patients with GD may have subclinical TED with extraocular muscle enlargement on imaging [6]. The prevalence and severity of TED may be declining in recent decades, a trend putatively related to the decline in smoking [2, 5]. The incidence of TED is approximately 5.5 times higher in women compared with men [7].

> **Summary for the Clinician**
> - There is a close temporal relationship between the onset of TED and hyperthyroidism due to GD.
> - The prevalence of TED in the United States is 0.25 % in the general population but 20–50 % among individuals with GD.

9.2   Pathophysiology

Recent decades have witnessed significant progress in our understanding of the pathophysiology of TED (Fig. 9.1). Enlargement of orbital soft tissues is the fundamental process that underlies most of the clinical manifestations of TED [8, 9]. Histopathological studies of the TED orbit reveal an extensive deposition of hyaluronan (a hydrophilic glycosaminoglycan) between muscle fibers leading to the enlargement of extraocular muscles, a widespread inflammatory infiltrate with associated interstitial edema, and an overabundance of cytokines [10, 11]. The principal cell type implicated in these changes is the orbital fibroblast (OF) [12–14]. These cells are aberrantly and robustly activated in TED. Once activated, they upregulate hyaluronan synthesis [15–22] and can differentiate into myofibroblasts, which play a role in wound healing and fibrosis, or adipocytes, which contribute to orbital fat expansion [13, 23–27]. Activated OFs also produce inflammatory cytokines, including potent T-cell chemoattractants, perpetuating the vicious cycle of inflammation [28–36]. Once T cells are recruited to the orbit, they interact with OFs leading to mutual activation [32]. Activated T cells then induce B-cell differentiation and activate monocytes and macrophages, further propagating the autoimmune and inflammatory process in TED [37]. Fibrocytes are bone-marrow-derived, fibroblast-like, progenitor cells that normally circulate in the peripheral blood but infiltrate the orbital tissues in GD patients [38, 39]. Within the orbit, fibrocytes behave like OFs and may play a role in TED pathogenesis [40].

The aberrant activation of OFs in TED likely involves at least two autoantigens, the thyrotropin receptor (TSHR) and insulin-like growth factor-1 receptor (IGF-1R). TSHR autoantibodies, a key player in the pathogenesis of GD, are detectable in up to 98 % of TED patients [41, 42]. Moreover, the titers of these autoantibodies positively correlate with TED activity and severity [42–46]. Accumulating evidence suggests that both TSHR and IGF-1R are upregulated in OFs and fibrocytes in TED [20, 47]. Further, IGF-1R-expressing T and B cells are more abundant in GD patients compared with controls [48, 49]. Immunizing mice with fragments of TSHR leads to the development of TSHR and IGF-1R autoantibodies and orbital changes that clinically, radiographically, and pathologically resemble those observed in humans with TED [50]. In vitro studies implicate both the TSHR and IGF-1R signaling pathways in the activation of OFs in TED, leading to hyaluronan synthesis, cytokine production, and fibroblast differentiation [20, 24, 25, 34, 43, 51–54]. These two receptors seem to form a physical and functional complex as immunofluorescence staining demonstrates co-localization of these receptors and blocking the IGF-1R pathway leads to attenuation of TSHR-mediated signaling as well [54–56]. Hence, these two autoantigens may work in a concerted fashion in the pathogenesis of TED.

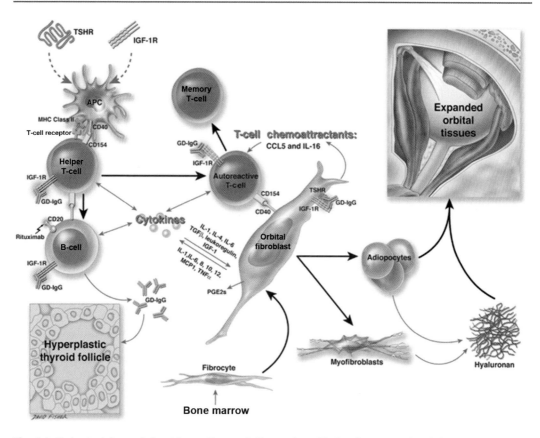

Fig. 9.1 Pathophysiology of thyroid eye disease. Self-tolerance to the autoantigens TSHR and IGF-1R is lost for unclear reasons. Antigen-presenting cells (*APC*) internalize TSHR and IGF-1R and present them to helper T cells, which become activated and may either induce B cells to produce autoantibodies (GD-IgGs) or become autoreactive T cells themselves. GD-IgGs interact with TSHR on thyroid epithelial cells, leading to follicular hyperplasia and hypertrophy. Autoreactive CD4 T cells travel to orbital tissues in response to T-cell chemoattractants and interact with orbital fibroblasts (OF), which leads to the mutual acti- vation of both cell types. Various inflammatory cytokines are secreted by T and B cells and OFs. Each of these cell types also overexpresses IGF-1R, which can interact with GD-IgGs, resulting in cellular activation. On the surface of OFs, IGF-1R and TSHR form a physical and functional complex that can interact with GD-IgGs. Some of the OFs in TED patients may be derived from infiltrating fibrocytes derived from the bone marrow. Activated OFs can differen- tiate into either adipocytes or myofibroblasts and have increased hyaluronan synthesis. Together, these processes lead to the expansion of orbital soft tissue in TED

Summary for the Clinician

- OFs are the principal effector cells impli- cated in orbital soft tissue enlargement in TED, through hyaluronan synthesis, cytokine production, and fibroblast differentiation.
- Fibrocytes are bone-marrow-derived, fibroblast-like, progenitor cells that may play a role in TED pathogenesis.
- The aberrant activation of OFs and fibrocytes in TED likely involves the autoantigens TSHR and IGF-1R.

9.3   Clinical Presentation and Diagnosis

The clinical manifestations of TED mostly arise from the enlargement of the orbital soft tissues. Confined within the rigid orbital walls, such tissue enlargement leads to increased intraorbital pres- sure, orbital congestion, mechanical tissue com- pression, and further inflammation [9]. Common clinical findings in TED include exophthalmos, eyelid retraction and lateral flare, lid lag on down gaze, lagophthalmos, and strabismus. The com- bined effects of exophthalmos and eyelid retraction can lead to corneal exposure, with severity ranging from epithelial erosions to impending perforation. When mechanical tissue compression occurs at the orbital apex and involves the optic nerve, a compressive optic neuropathy (CON) occurs. The most useful clinical signs in diagnosing CON are decreased visual acuity, dyschromatopsia, relative afferent papillary defect (unless the condition is bilateral), and optic disc swelling or atrophy [57–59]. Visual field defects have been reported in approximately 71 % of patients with CON, but they are not specific for CON [58, 60–64].

If the clinical history and exam suggest a diagnosis of TED, thyroid status should be assessed using thyroid function tests (thyroid hormones T3 and free T4 and thyroid-stimulating hormone). Thyroid-stimulating immunoglobulin titers should be obtained, as this autoantibody is present in up to 98 % of TED patients [4, 42]. Abnormalities in these studies would support the clinical diagnosis, but false negatives may occur, especially in long-standing TED. Orbital imaging is informative but not necessary in establishing the diagnosis. Orbital computed tomography (CT) is the imaging modality of choice. The principle advantage of CT is its precise visualization of the orbital bony architecture including the orbital apex. Orbital CT is also indispensable in surgical planning for orbital decompression. Magnetic resonance imaging may show soft tissue inflammatory changes in active TED, but does not provide sufficient details about the bony anatomy [65]. Similarly, while ultrasonography can be used to measure the caliber and internal reflectivity of the extraocular muscles, it provides no information about the bony structures and is highly dependent on technician expertise [65].

TED can be classified into three categories based on the severity of subjective symptoms and objective signs (i.e., the European Group on Graves' Orbitopathy classification): mild, moderate-to-severe, and sight-threatening disease (Table 9.1) [66]. Most cases of TED are mild and self-limited [5, 67]. Only 15–25 % of these patients progress to more severe disease [4]. Up to one third of TED patients have moderate-to-severe disease on presentation [7, 68]. Sight-threatening disease affects 4–8.6 % of TED

Table 9.1 European Group on Graves' Orbitopathy (EUGOGO) severity classification

Sight-threatening	CON and/or corneal breakdown. Immediate intervention is warranted.
Moderate to severe	No sight-threatening TED. One or more of: lid retraction ≥2 mm, moderate-or-severe soft tissue involvement, exophthalmos ≥3 mm above normal for race and gender, inconstant or constant diplopia. Disease has sufficient impact on daily life to justify the risks of immunosuppression (if active) or surgical intervention (if inactive).
Mild	One or more of: minimal lid retraction <2 mm, mild soft tissue involvement, exophthalmos <3 mm above normal for race and gender, transient or no diplopia, and corneal exposure responsive to lubricants. Only minor impact on daily life, insufficient to justify immunosuppressive or surgical treatment.

patients [7, 57, 69]. Another severity classification system for TED is the NO SPECS classification, which generates a global score for disease severity (Table 9.2) [70]. TED can also be classified based on disease activity. There are two phases of TED: an active phase lasting from 6 to 24 months, followed by an inactive phase, where the disease plateaus and remains quiescent [71]. Active TED presents with evidence of periorbital soft tissue inflammation. The clinical activity score (CAS) uses these features of inflammation to estimate the activity of disease (Table 9.3) [72]. The VISA classification system assesses for both disease severity and activity [73].

> **Summary for the Clinician**
> - Common clinical findings of TED include exophthalmos, eyelid malposition, and strabismus.
> - Clinical history and exam form the basis of diagnosis for TED, but abnormalities in thyroid function and immunological tests would support the diagnosis.
> - Orbital CT is the imaging modality of choice for TED.
> - Various severity and activity grading systems exist for TED.

Table 9.2 NO SPECS classification

Class	Grade
0	*N*o physical signs or symptoms
I	*O*nly signs (eyelid retraction)
II	*S*oft tissue involvement 0, absent; a, minimal; b, moderate; c marked
III	*P*roptosis 0, absent; a, minimal; b, moderate; c, marked
IV	*E*xtraocular muscle signs 0, absent; a, limitation in extremes of gaze; b, evident restriction; c, fixation of globe(s)
V	*C*orneal involvement 0, absent; a, stippling; b, ulceration; c, clouding, necrosis, perforation
VI	*S*ight loss 0, VA better than 20/25; a, VA 20/30 to 20/60; b, VA 20/70 to 20/150; c, VA 20/200 or worse

Table 9.3 Clinical activity score

Pain	Painful feeling behind globe within the last 4 weeks Pain on attempted gaze within the last 4 weeks
Redness	Redness of eyelid(s) Redness of conjunctiva
Swelling	Chemosis Swelling of eyelid(s) Swelling of carbuncle Increase of proptosis of ≥ 2 mm within the last 1–3 months
Impaired function	Decrease in visual acuity of ≥ 1 line(s) on the Snellen chart within the last 1–3 months Decrease in eye movements of $\geq 5°$ within the last 1–3 months

One point is given for each item using a binary scale. The sum of points is the clinical activity score

9.4 Management

9.4.1 Risk Factor Modifications

Three main modifiable risk factors are associated with the development of de novo or worsening TED: smoking, diabetes mellitus, and dysthyroidism. Smoking is the most important modifiable risk factor for TED [74–76]. Patients with Graves' disease who smoke are more likely to develop TED [5, 75, 76] than nonsmokers, and patients with TED who smoke tend to have more severe disease and are less responsive to therapy [76–78]. Therefore, smoking cessation should be discussed upon diagnosis and remain a critical element of management for all patients with TED. Diabetes mellitus is an important risk factor associated with the development of CON. Patients with CON are more likely to be diabetic, and TED patients with diabetes mellitus are more likely to develop more severe CON with worse visual prognosis [60, 69, 79]. Diabetic microvasculopathy in the optic nerve may sensitize it to compressive pressure [79]. No studies have established a dose-response relationship between glycemic control and the development of CON. Nevertheless, upon diagnosing TED in a diabetic patient, it would be prudent to alert the primary care provider of this diagnosis and emphasize to the patient the importance of glycemic control.

Persistent dysthyroidism is another modifiable risk factor for more severe TED [80]. The restoration and maintenance of euthyroidism is associated with improvement of TED and should be the goal in every patient with TED [5]. Three treatment modalities are used to normalize thyroid function: radioablation using iodine–131 (RAI), antithyroid medication, and total or partial thyroidectomy. RAI therapy is associated with the development or worsening of TED in 15–35 % of patients [81–83], possibly related to the destruction of thyroid tissue, release of thyroid autoantigens, and subsequent exacerbation of the autoimmune reaction [84]. This adverse effect of RAI may be prevented or reduced by concomitant administration of low-dose (0.2 mg/kg/day) systemic oral glucocorticoids beginning 1 week prior to RAI and gradually tapered over 6 weeks following RAI [75, 82]. For patients with active TED and moderate-to-severe or sight-threatening TED, other treatment modalities such as antithyroid medication or thyroidectomy should be considered, as neither has been shown to affect the course of TED [85].

Summary for the Clinician
- Smoking cessation is of paramount importance for all patients with GD and TED.
- TED patients with diabetes mellitus are at increased risk to develop CON.

- Euthyroidism should be achieved and maintained in all patients with TED.
- RAI should be given with concomitant low-dose systemic glucocorticoids to prevent new development or exacerbation of TED.
- RAI should be avoided in patients with active TED and moderate-to-severe or sight-threatening TED.

Summary for the Clinician
- Conservative measures are the mainstay of treatment for mild TED.
- Patients with mild TED could be offered a course of selenium supplementation.

9.4.3 Moderate-to-Severe or Sight-Threatening Disease

The therapeutic approach for moderate-to-severe or sight-threatening TED depends on the activity of disease. If the disease is active, systemic glucocorticoids should be the first line of therapy with or without adjunctive low-dose external beam radiotherapy. The goal of treatment is to abort or shorten the acute inflammatory phase. If the disease is sight-threatening and is refractory to systemic glucocorticoids, then urgent orbital decompression surgery should be performed. If the disease is inactive, neither systemic glucocorticoids nor orbital radiotherapy (ORT) tend to be effective [90]. Instead, rehabilitative surgery may be considered.

9.4.3.1 Active Disease
Systemic Glucocorticoids
The current first line of therapy for active moderate-to-severe and sight-threatening TED is systemic glucocorticoids [66, 90]. In addition to having anti-inflammatory and immuno-suppressive properties [91], glucocorticoids can also decrease hyaluronan synthesis by OFs [92]. Over the past two decades, five randomized controlled trials have shown that glucocorticoids are more effective when given intravenously than by mouth in treating moderate-to-severe and sight-threatening TED (response rates of approximately 80 and 60 %, respectively) [91]. The intravenous route of administration is also associated with fewer side effects (side effect rates of 56 and 85 %, respectively) [66, 93]. Therefore, intravenous glucocorticoids are currently the first line of therapy for active TED.

9.4.2 Mild Disease

Most cases of TED are mild, and most mild cases of TED improve spontaneously [5, 67, 86]. Nevertheless, even mild TED can have significant impact on patients' quality of life with disturbing symptoms [87]. The mainstay of treatment for mild TED is to use conservative measures to alleviate these symptoms [88]. Ocular surface lubricating artificial tears and ointment with or without moisture chamber at night time is used to address symptoms of exposure. Cold compresses, low sodium diet, and head elevation during sleep may decrease dependent orbital edema [1, 66, 75]. Prisms or patching can be helpful for symptomatic diplopia.

Recent evidence suggests that patients with mild TED should be offered selenium supplementation upon diagnosis [88]. Selenium is a trace element incorporated into serum seleno-protein P, which acts as an antioxidant and has immunomodulatory effects [4, 75]. In a randomized controlled trial, treatment of patients with mild TED using sodium selenite (100 mg twice daily by mouth) for 6 months was associated with lower rate of progression to more severe TED and improvement in ocular involvement and quality of life compared to placebo [89]. Most of the patients in this study were from marginally selenium-deficient areas, so whether selenium supplementation would be as beneficial for those living in selenium-sufficient areas remains to be established.

The optimal regimen of IV glucocorticoids for TED has not been established. The commonly used regimen is 12 infusions of methylprednisolone, 500 mg weekly for 6 weeks, followed by 250 mg weekly for 6 weeks [88, 94]. The cumulative dose should not exceed 8 g in each 12-week treatment course, and infusions should not be given on consecutive or alternate days. For patients with sight-threatening disease, especially CON, IV methylprednisolone high-dose pulse therapy is typically given: 1 g daily for three consecutive days, repeated in the second week if necessary [95]. If the response is sufficient, an oral prednisone taper is initiated upon completion of pulse therapy. Immediate orbital decompression surgery appears to have no advantage over initial pulse therapy for CON [96]. Orbital decompression surgery should be performed in cases of severe orbital congestion, if the response to pulse therapy is insufficient or if glucocorticoids are contraindicated [88, 97, 98].

Systemic glucocorticoids therapy has a multitude of adverse effects. A meta-analysis of 1,461 patients with moderate-to-severe TED treated with IV glucocorticoids reported a morbidity and mortality rate of 6.5 and 0.6 %, respectively [91]. The mortalities were due to acute liver failure and cerebrovascular or cardiovascular events [88, 99–103]. These serious systemic side effects appear to be dose related, as nearly all of these patients received a cumulative dose of 8 g or more when the fatal adverse event occurred [88]. Systemic risk factors such as uncontrolled hypertension, uncontrolled diabetes mellitus, cardiac arrhythmias, hypokalemia, or liver dysfunction including a history of viral or autoimmune hepatitis may constitute contraindications to systemic glucocorticoids therapy [99, 100, 102, 104, 105]. During each course of IV glucocorticoids therapy, patients should be carefully monitored for the development of side effects.

> **Summary for the Clinician**
> - The first line of therapy for moderate-to-severe TED is 12 infusions of IV methylprednisolone, 500 mg weekly for 6 weeks, followed by 250 mg weekly for 6 weeks.
> - The first line of therapy for CON is IV methylprednisolone pulse therapy, 1 g daily for three consecutive days, and repeated in the second week if necessary, followed by oral prednisone taper.
> - For CON, if the response to pulse therapy is insufficient, emergent orbital decompression surgery is indicated.
> - Patients must be carefully assessed for systemic risk factors prior to initiating glucocorticoids therapy and followed closely during treatment for the development of side effects.

Orbital Radiotherapy

Low-dose external beam ORT is an adjunctive treatment for TED but its efficacy remains uncertain [106]. The effects may be mediated by interfering with the nitric oxide pathway [90, 107]. ORT can also impair the function of lymphocytes that infiltrate the orbit [106] and reduce the capability of OFs to synthesize hyaluronan [108]. Similar to glucocorticoids therapy, ORT appears to offer most utility in active TED. Whereas the effects of glucocorticoids therapy are immediate in onset but short-lasting, the effects of ORT are delayed, often taking weeks to months for the maximal clinical effect. For this reason, ORT is typically not used as the initial treatment, but rather as an adjunctive therapy to maintain remission during glucocorticoids taper, or in patients who cannot tolerate or have insufficient response to glucocorticoids therapy [108]. Whether or not the combination therapy of IV glucocorticoids with ORT truly offers additional benefit compared with IV glucocorticoids alone remains to be established [4, 93, 97, 98, 109, 110].

ORT with modern standardized protocols is well tolerated and relatively safe [111, 112]. The conventional regimen is to deliver a total of 20 Gy, divided over ten fractions, aimed at the retrobulbar tissue of each orbit [113]. Lower dosing regimens may have similar response rates and be better tolerated [111, 114, 115]. Randomized controlled studies are needed to assess not only the efficacy of ORT as adjuvant therapy but also its optimal regimen. Potential side effects of ORT include skin erythema, temporary focal alopecia, conjunctival injection, cataract, radiation retinopathy, and optic neuropathy [110–112, 114]. Uncontrolled hypertension and diabetes mellitus are contraindications to ORT due to an increased risk of de novo or deteriorating retinopathy [111]. Finally, there is a theoretical cumulative lifetime risk of up to 1.2 % of developing secondary malignancies in the radiated field after low-dose ORT [111, 112, 116]. Therefore, even though no such cases have yet been reported, ORT should be restricted to TED patients older than 35 years of age due to the long latency of these tumors.

Summary for the Clinician
- ORT can be used as an adjunctive therapy for active TED with IV glucocorticoids as the first line of therapy.
- The clinical effects of ORT tend to be more delayed than those of IV glucocorticoids.
- The conventional protocol is to deliver a total of 20 Gy external beam radiation divided over ten fractions, but lower doses may be effective.
- Uncontrolled hypertension and diabetes mellitus are contraindications to ORT due to an increased risk of retinopathy.
- ORT should be restricted to patients older than 35 years of age due to a theoretical risk of secondary ORT-induced malignancy.

Novel Therapeutic Agents

Lacking in our current therapeutic armamentarium for TED are disease-modifying agents that alter the underlying pathologic process. Various novel biologic agents have been purported to be beneficial in treating moderate-to-severe TED in small, uncontrolled studies [117–122]. Yet, none have shown definitive advantage over IV glucocorticoids with or without ORT in long-term disease outcome [117–122]. Several randomized controlled trials are being conducted to assess the efficacy of three of these agents: rituximab, an IGF-1R monoclonal antibody, and zidovudine [4, 119].

Rituximab is a CD20+ B-cell-depleting monoclonal antibody. It is one of the most promising disease-modifying agents for TED [123]. Rituximab blocks B-cell proliferation and maturation (Fig. 9.1) and has been shown in several retrospective reports and open-label studies to be effective in treating moderate-to-severe and sight-threatening TED [124–132]. To date, 43 patients with TED have been treated with rituximab; disease became inactive in 91 % of these patients [123]. Importantly, the treatment effect of rituximab may occur as rapidly as within 1–3 h, making it an attractive option for sight-threatening TED [125]. Side effects have been reported in one third of the patients, most of which are infusion-related reactions [123]. Rituximab is currently reserved for patients who do not tolerate IV glucocorticoids or have disease that is refractory to conventional therapy. Three randomized controlled trials are underway to evaluate the efficacy of rituximab in treating TED.

Summary for the Clinician
- Rituximab is a CD20+ B-cell-depleting monoclonal antibody that can block B-cell proliferation and maturation.
- Using rituximab to treat moderate-to-severe and sight-threatening TED has shown a 91 % response rate so far in uncontrolled studies.
- Large-scale randomized controlled trials to evaluate the efficacy of rituximab in treating TED are underway.

Urgent Surgical Management

Surgical management of TED is typically reserved for inactive disease. However, if sight-threatening TED is refractory to medical therapy, or if IV glucocorticoids are contraindicated or poorly tolerated, then urgent surgical management is indicated, even if the disease is active [133].

Orbital Decompression Surgery

The goal of orbital decompression surgery is to remove parts of the bony orbital walls and/or orbital fat, thereby allowing the enlarged and congested orbital soft tissues to expand into new effective orbital space, relieving intraorbital pressure [133, 134]. For patients with CON, if there is insufficient response after 3 days of IV methylprednisolone pulse therapy, urgent surgical decompression should be performed. The decompression should focus on the posteromedial orbit and the orbital apex and is shown to have a rapid and beneficial effect on vision [135–139]. Specifically, the deep medial wall including the middle and posterior ethmoidal air cells, the posteromedial orbital floor, and the posterior infraorbital strut are removed [140]. The deep lateral wall can also be decompressed to further relieve compression of the posterior orbit [4].

For patients with significant exophthalmos leading to severe exposure keratopathy, various approaches to orbital decompression can be used. The desired extent of exophthalmos reduction dictates the amount of orbital fat and the number of orbital walls to be removed. Orbital fat resection should be considered in all patients undergoing decompression. Resection of orbital fat alone can lead to an average reduction of 1.8 mm in exophthalmos [113, 141], as well as intraorbital pressure reduction [113, 135, 137, 141–145]. If CON is not present, the lateral wall is often the first choice of orbital walls to be removed, as this is associated with a lower risk of postoperative diplopia compared with medial wall or orbital floor decompression [146–148]. Traditionally, the zygoma from the frontozygomatic suture to just above the zygomatic arch is removed [140, 149, 150]. A modified technique, the deep lateral wall approach, removes the lateral wall and the marrow of the sphenoid extending to the orbital fissures and anteriorly to the orbital rim [135, 151]. This technique allows posterior axial displacement of the globe rather than horizontal or inferior displacement, thereby reducing the risk of postoperative diplopia [135, 146].

Decompression of the medial wall is most commonly performed endoscopically or externally using the transcaruncular approach. The osteotomy extends superiorly to the level of the anterior and posterior ethmoidal arteries, anteriorly to the posterior lacrimal crest, and inferiorly to the bony maxilloethmoidal strut [140]. Though rarely necessary decompression of the orbital floor can also be performed endoscopically or using a transconjunctival approach through the inferior fornix [136, 152–155]. The osteotomy extends anteriorly to the orbital rim, posteriorly to the posterior wall of the maxillary sinus, laterally to the inferior orbital fissure, and medially to the medial orbital wall. Care is taken to preserve the infraorbital canal and neurovascular bundle. Depending on the level of exophthalmos, a "balanced" decompression (medial and lateral walls) or a "three-wall decompression" (medial and lateral walls and orbital floor) may be performed [140, 151, 156].

The most common adverse effect of orbital decompression surgery is de novo or worsening diplopia [157, 158], which occurs in 10–30 % of patients [159]. This is mostly caused by the displacement of the rectus muscles away from the orbital axis [160–162]. The risk of postoperative diplopia is significantly higher with medial wall and orbital floor decompression (up to two third of patients) compared with lateral wall decompression (2–7 % of patients) [146–148]. Leaving the maxilloethmoidal strut intact reduces the risk of postoperative diplopia [163]. Medial wall decompression may also lead to sinusitis and cerebrospinal fluid leak. Orbital floor decompression carries a risk of hypoesthesia of the cheek and lower eyelid due to damage to the infraorbital nerve. Other potential complications of orbital decompression may be caused by intraoperative damage to important anatomical structures such as the optic nerve or rectus muscles. Stereotactic guidance during decompression surgery may be helpful in allowing precise localization and visualization of the extent of bone removal in real time, which may decrease the risk of iatrogenic injury to important anatomical structures [108, 164].

Temporizing Eyelid Procedures

Patients with severe exposure keratopathy due to exophthalmos and eyelid retraction may need to undergo emergent eyelid retractor recession with or without temporary suture tarsorrhaphy in addition to orbital decompression to protect the ocular surface. The eyelid retractor recession procedures will be discussed in detail in the next section. These patients should also receive intensive topical lubrication with moisture chamber. The usage of botulinum toxin has been described for upper eyelid retraction in active TED as a temporizing measure [165–167]. However, its effect is limited, delayed (by up to 48 h), and unpredictable [4]. Further, there is a risk that the adjacent superior rectus could be inadvertently affected by the toxin, leading to reduced Bell's phenomenon, thereby exacerbating corneal exposure [4].

Summary for Clinicians
- If sight-threatening TED is insufficiently responsive to IV glucocorticoids, then urgent surgical management is indicated.
- To treat CON, surgical decompression needs to focus on the posteromedial orbit, relieving compression at the orbital apex.
- Orbital decompression surgery to reduce exophthalmos can involve orbital fat resection and removal of parts of the lateral wall, medial wall, and, rarely, orbital floor.
- The most common adverse effect of surgical decompression is postoperative diplopia, which is more common after medial wall and orbital floor decompression than lateral wall decompression.
- Patients with severe exposure keratopathy in the active phase may also require eyelid retractor recession with or without suture tarsorrhaphy.

9.4.3.2 Inactive Disease
Surgical rehabilitation may be indicated for inactive TED with significant residual cosmetic and functional changes. Prior to rehabilitative surgery, TED must be nonprogressive for at least 6 months, and the patient should have been stably maintained in euthyroidism. The first step of surgical rehabilitation is orbital decompression for significant exophthalmos. The second step is

extraocular muscle surgery for ocular misalignment, performed at least 3 months after orbital decompression to allow the globe to settle in its new position, and after at least 6 months of stable alignment measurements. The last step is eyelid surgery for eyelid malposition, performed at least 2 months after extraocular muscle surgery. This is because the vertical extraocular muscles can impact upper and lower eyelid positioning.

Orbital Decompression Surgery
The principles of orbital decompression in inactive TED are similar to those for active disease, as discussed in the previous section.

Extraocular Muscle Surgery
The enlargement and fibrosis of extraocular muscles in TED leads to their decreased elasticity while preserving contractility. This results in restrictive strabismus, which should be repaired by extraocular muscle recession. The inferior rectus is the most commonly affected muscle, followed by the medial rectus. Inferior rectus recession may lead to worsened lower eyelid retraction. Recession in general can worsen exophthalmos. Therefore, if both orbital decompression and extraocular muscle recessions are indicated, one should aim for overcorrection of the former in anticipation for worsened exophthalmos after the latter. Due to the complexity of the ocular misalignment in TED, the overarching goal of surgery is to restore binocular single vision in the primary position at distance and near [133]. Residual diplopia may persist in other positions of gaze. Numerous operations may be required to achieve satisfactory results.

Eyelid Surgery
Eyelid retraction repair is generally indicated for eyelid retraction of more than 1 mm, lateral flare, or asymmetry between the palpebral apertures [133]. Upper eyelid retraction may be caused by sympathetic stimulation or fibrosis of the levator palpebrae superioris or Muller's muscle [168]. Repair requires recession of one or both of these muscles through an anterior (eyelid crease incision) or posterior (conjunctival) approach, respectively. Disinsertion of the lateral horn of

the levator aponeurosis from the tarsus can correct lateral flare. Upper eyelid retraction repair has an average success rate of 70–80 % [133].

Lower eyelid retraction may occur due to fibrosis of the lower eyelid retractors or after inferior rectus recession during extraocular muscle surgery. Repair is typically performed through a posterior (conjunctival) approach, but minimally invasive techniques such as en gY lysis of the lower eyelid retractors have been described [169]. The lower eyelid retractors are disinserted from the tarsus, and a spacer is placed in between to lengthen the lower eyelid. Various organic and synthetic spacer materials have been used [170–178]. The amount of desired lower eyelid elevation determines the size of the spacer. The effect of lower eyelid lengthening can be enhanced by a lateral tarsal strip procedure and/or a tarsorrhaphy [172].

Another indication for eyelid surgery in TED is dermatochalasis and increased preaponeurotic and subdermal fat leading to the appearance of bulging eyelids. Blepharoplasty with fat excision can be performed for both upper and lower eyelids. Skin excision in the lower eyelid should be conservative as excessive excision may lead to lower eyelid retraction or ectropion [155]. In patients who have prolapsing fat but without excess skin, fat excision can also be performed through a transconjunctival approach without blepharoplasty.

Summary for Clinicians

- TED must be stable and nonprogressive for at least 6 months prior to surgical rehabilitation.
- TED rehabilitative surgery should be performed in the following sequence: orbital decompression, extraocular muscle surgery, and eyelid surgery.
- TED-associated restrictive strabismus should be corrected by extraocular muscle recession.
- Upper eyelid retraction involves recession of the upper eyelid retractors. Lower eyelid retraction repair requires both recession of the lower eyelid retractors and the insertion of a spacer graft.

Compliance with Ethical Requirements Shannon S. Joseph and Raymond S. Douglas declare that they have no conflict of interest.

No human or animal studies were carried out by the authors for this article.

References

1. Dolman PJ. Evaluating Graves' orbitopathy. Best Pract Res Clin Endocrinol Metab. 2012;26(3):229–48.
2. Lazarus JH. Epidemiology of Graves' orbitopathy (GO) and relationship with thyroid disease. Best Pract Res Clin Endocrinol Metab. 2012;26(3):273–9.
3. Marcocci C, Bartalena L, Bogazzi F, Panicucci M, Pinchera A. Studies on the occurrence of ophthalmopathy in Graves' disease. Acta Endocrinol (Copenh). 1989;120(4):473–8.
4. Verity DH, Rose GE. Acute thyroid eye disease (TED): principles of medical and surgical management. Eye (Lond). 2013;27(3):308–19.
5. Tanda ML, Piantanida E, Liparulo L, Veronesi G, Lai A, Sassi L, et al. Prevalence and natural history of Graves' orbitopathy in a large series of patients with newly diagnosed graves' hyperthyroidism seen at a single center. J Clin Endocrinol Metab. 2013;98(4):1443–9.
6. Enzmann DR, Donaldson SS, Kriss JP. Appearance of Graves' disease on orbital computed tomography. J Comput Assist Tomogr. 1979;3(6):815–9.
7. Bartley GB. The epidemiologic characteristics and clinical course of ophthalmopathy associated with autoimmune thyroid disease in Olmsted County, Minnesota. Trans Am Ophthalmol Soc. 1994;92:477–588.
8. Forbes G, Gorman CA, Brennan MD, Gehring DG, Ilstrup DM, Earnest F. Ophthalmopathy of Graves' disease: computerized volume measurements of the orbital fat and muscle. AJNR Am J Neuroradiol. 1986;7(4):651–6.
9. Bahn RS. Graves' ophthalmopathy. N Engl J Med. 2010;362(8):726–38.
10. Smith TJ, Bahn RS, Gorman CA. Connective tissue, glycosaminoglycans, and diseases of the thyroid. Endocr Rev. 1989;10(3):366–91.
11. Hufnagel TJ, Hickey WF, Cobbs WH, Jakobiec FA, Iwamoto T, Eagle RC. Immunohistochemical and ultrastructural studies on the exenterated orbital tissues of a patient with Graves' disease. Ophthalmology. 1984;91(11):1411–9.
12. Smith RS, Smith TJ, Blieden TM, Phipps RP. Fibroblasts as sentinel cells. Synthesis of chemokines and regulation of inflammation. Am J Pathol. 1997;151(2):317–22.
13. Smith TJ, Koumas L, Gagnon A, Bell A, Sempowski GD, Phipps RP, et al. Orbital fibroblast heterogeneity may determine the clinical presentation of thyroid-associated ophthalmopathy. J Clin Endocrinol Metab. 2002;87(1):385–92.

14. Smith TJ, Tsai CC, Shih MJ, Tsui S, Chen B, Han R, et al. Unique attributes of orbital fibroblasts and global alterations in IGF-1 receptor signaling could explain thyroid-associated ophthalmopathy. Thyroid. 2008;18(9):983–8.

15. Korducki JM, Loftus SJ, Bahn RS. Stimulation of glycosaminoglycan production in cultured human retroocular fibroblasts. Invest Ophthalmol Vis Sci. 1992;33(6):2037–42.

16. Smith TJ, Wang HS, Evans CH. Leukoregulin is a potent inducer of hyaluronan synthesis in cultured human orbital fibroblasts. Am J Physiol. 1995;268(2 Pt 1):C382–8.

17. Cao HJ, Wang HS, Zhang Y, Lin HY, Phipps RP, Smith TJ. Activation of human orbital fibroblasts through CD40 engagement results in a dramatic induction of hyaluronan synthesis and prostaglandin endoperoxide H synthase-2 expression. Insights into potential pathogenic mechanisms of thyroid-associated ophthalmopathy. J Biol Chem. 1998;273(45):29615–25.

18. Kaback LA, Smith TJ. Expression of hyaluronan synthase messenger ribonucleic acids and their induction by interleukin-1beta in human orbital fibroblasts: potential insight into the molecular pathogenesis of thyroid-associated ophthalmopathy. J Clin Endocrinol Metab. 1999;84(11):4079–84.

19. Han R, Smith TJ. T helper type 1 and type 2 cytokines exert divergent influence on the induction of prostaglandin E2 and hyaluronan synthesis by interleukin-1beta in orbital fibroblasts: implications for the pathogenesis of thyroid-associated ophthalmopathy. Endocrinology. 2006;147(1):13–9.

20. Smith TJ, Hoa N. Immunoglobulins from patients with Graves' disease induce hyaluronan synthesis in their orbital fibroblasts through the self-antigen, insulin-like growth factor-I receptor. J Clin Endocrinol Metab. 2004;89(10):5076–80.

21. Krieger CC, Gershengorn MC. A modified ELISA accurately measures secretion of high molecular weight hyaluronan (HA) by Graves' disease orbital cells. Endocrinology. 2014;155(2):627–34.

22. Tan GH, Dutton CM, Bahn RS. Interleukin-1 (IL-1) receptor antagonist and soluble IL-1 receptor inhibit IL-1-induced glycosaminoglycan production in cultured human orbital fibroblasts from patients with Graves' ophthalmopathy. J Clin Endocrinol Metab. 1996;81(2):449–52.

23. Sorisky A, Pardasani D, Gagnon A, Smith TJ. Evidence of adipocyte differentiation in human orbital fibroblasts in primary culture. J Clin Endocrinol Metab. 1996;81(9):3428–31.

24. Valyasevi RW, Erickson DZ, Harteneck DA, Dutton CM, Heufelder AE, Jyonouchi SC, et al. Differentiation of human orbital preadipocyte fibroblasts induces expression of functional thyrotropin receptor. J Clin Endocrinol Metab. 1999;84(7):2557–62.

25. Valyasevi RW, Harteneck DA, Dutton CM, Bahn RS. Stimulation of adipogenesis, peroxisome proliferator-activated receptor-gamma (PPARgamma), and thyrotropin receptor by PPARgamma agonist in human orbital preadipocyte fibroblasts. J Clin Endocrinol Metab. 2002;87(5):2352–8.

26. Koumas L, Smith TJ, Feldon S, Blumberg N, Phipps RP. Thy-1 expression in human fibroblast subsets defines myofibroblastic or lipofibroblastic phenotypes. Am J Pathol. 2003;163(4):1291–300.

27. Feldon SE, O'Loughlin CW, Ray DM, Landskroner-Eiger S, Seweryniak KE, Phipps RP. Activated human T lymphocytes express cyclooxygenase-2 and produce proadipogenic prostaglandins that drive human orbital fibroblast differentiation to adipocytes. Am J Pathol. 2006;169(4):1183–93.

28. Han R, Tsui S, Smith TJ. Up-regulation of prostaglandin E2 synthesis by interleukin-1beta in human orbital fibroblasts involves coordinate induction of prostaglandin-endoperoxide H synthase-2 and glutathione-dependent prostaglandin E2 synthase expression. J Biol Chem. 2002;277(19):16355–64.

29. Wang HS, Cao HJ, Winn VD, Rezanka LJ, Frobert Y, Evans CH, et al. Leukoregulin induction of prostaglandin-endoperoxide H synthase-2 in human orbital fibroblasts. An in vitro model for connective tissue inflammation. J Biol Chem. 1996;271(37):22718–28.

30. Cao HJ, Smith TJ. Leukoregulin upregulation of prostaglandin endoperoxide H synthase-2 expression in human orbital fibroblasts. Am J Physiol. 1999;277(6 Pt 1):C1075–85.

31. Young DA, Evans CH, Smith TJ. Leukoregulin induction of protein expression in human orbital fibroblasts: evidence for anatomical site-restricted cytokine-target cell interactions. Proc Natl Acad Sci U S A. 1998;95(15):8904–9.

32. Hwang CJ, Afifiyan N, Sand D, Naik V, Said J, Pollock SJ, et al. Orbital fibroblasts from patients with thyroid-associated ophthalmopathy overexpress CD40: CD154 hyperinduces IL-6, IL-8, and MCP-1. Invest Ophthalmol Vis Sci. 2009;50(5):2262–8.

33. Sciaky D, Brazer W, Center DM, Cruikshank WW, Smith TJ. Cultured human fibroblasts express constitutive IL-16 mRNA: cytokine induction of active IL-16 protein synthesis through a caspase-3-dependent mechanism. J Immunol. 2000;164(7):3806–14.

34. Pritchard J, Han R, Horst N, Cruikshank WW, Smith TJ. Immunoglobulin activation of T cell chemoattractant expression in fibroblasts from patients with Graves' disease is mediated through the insulin-like growth factor I receptor pathway. J Immunol. 2003;170(12):6348–54.

35. Cao HJ, Han R, Smith TJ. Robust induction of PGHS-2 by IL-1 in orbital fibroblasts results from low levels of IL-1 receptor antagonist expression. Am J Physiol Cell Physiol. 2003;284(6):C1429–37.

36. Heufelder AE, Bahn RS. Modulation of Graves' orbital fibroblast proliferation by cytokines and glucocorticoid receptor agonists. Invest Ophthalmol Vis Sci. 1994;35(1):120–7.

37. Grewal IS, Flavell RA. The role of CD40 ligand in costimulation and T-cell activation. Immunol Rev. 1996;153:85–106.
38. Douglas RS, Afifiyan NF, Hwang CJ, Chong K, Haider U, Richards P, et al. Increased generation of fibrocytes in thyroid-associated ophthalmopathy. J Clin Endocrinol Metab. 2010;95(1):430–8.
39. Smith TJ, Padovani-Claudio DA, Lu Y, Raychaudhuri N, Fernando R, Atkins S, et al. Fibroblasts expressing the thyrotropin receptor overarch thyroid and orbit in Graves' disease. J Clin Endocrinol Metab. 2011;96(12):3827–37.
40. Hong KM, Belperio JA, Keane MP, Burdick MD, Strieter RM. Differentiation of human circulating fibrocytes as mediated by transforming growth factor-beta and peroxisome proliferator-activated receptor gamma. J Biol Chem. 2007;282(31):22910–20.
41. Weetman AP. Graves' disease. N Engl J Med. 2000;343(17):1236–48.
42. Ponto KA, Kanitz M, Olivo PD, Pitz S, Pfeiffer N, Kahaly GJ. Clinical relevance of thyroid-stimulating immunoglobulins in graves' ophthalmopathy. Ophthalmology. 2011;118(11):2279–85.
43. Gerding MN, van der Meer JW, Broenink M, Bakker O, Wiersinga WM, Prummel MF. Association of thyrotrophin receptor antibodies with the clinical features of Graves' ophthalmopathy. Clin Endocrinol (Oxf). 2000;52(3):267–71.
44. Eckstein AK, Plicht M, Lax H, Hirche H, Quadbeck B, Mann K, et al. Clinical results of anti-inflammatory therapy in Graves' ophthalmopathy and association with thyroidal autoantibodies. Clin Endocrinol (Oxf). 2004;61(5):612–8.
45. Eckstein AK, Plicht M, Lax H, Neuhauser M, Mann K, Lederbogen S, et al. Thyrotropin receptor autoantibodies are independent risk factors for Graves' ophthalmopathy and help to predict severity and outcome of the disease. J Clin Endocrinol Metab. 2006;91(9):3464–70.
46. Lytton SD, Ponto KA, Kanitz M, Matheis N, Kohn LD, Kahaly GJ. A novel thyroid stimulating immunoglobulin bioassay is a functional indicator of activity and severity of Graves' orbitopathy. J Clin Endocrinol Metab. 2010;95(5):2123–31.
47. Wakelkamp IM, Bakker O, Baldeschi L, Wiersinga WM, Prummel MF. TSH-R expression and cytokine profile in orbital tissue of active vs. inactive Graves' ophthalmopathy patients. Clin Endocrinol (Oxf). 2003;58(3):280–7.
48. Douglas RS, Gianoukakis AG, Kamat S, Smith TJ. Aberrant expression of the insulin-like growth factor-1 receptor by T cells from patients with Graves' disease may carry functional consequences for disease pathogenesis. J Immunol. 2007;178(5):3281–7.
49. Douglas RS, Naik V, Hwang CJ, Afifiyan NF, Gianoukakis AG, Sand D, et al. B cells from patients with Graves' disease aberrantly express the IGF-1 receptor: implications for disease pathogenesis. J Immunol. 2008;181(8):5768–74.
50. Moshkelgosha S, So PW, Deasy N, Diaz-Cano S, Banga JP. Cutting edge: retrobulbar inflammation, adipogenesis, and acute orbital congestion in a pre-clinical female mouse model of Graves' orbitopathy induced by thyrotropin receptor plasmid-in vivo electroporation. Endocrinology. 2013;154(9):3008–15.
51. Jyonouchi SC, Valyasevi RW, Harteneck DA, Dutton CM, Bahn RS. Interleukin-6 stimulates thyrotropin receptor expression in human orbital preadipocyte fibroblasts from patients with Graves' ophthalmopathy. Thyroid. 2001;11(10):929–34.
52. Starkey KJ, Janezic A, Jones G, Jordan N, Baker G, Ludgate M. Adipose thyrotrophin receptor expression is elevated in Graves' and thyroid eye diseases ex vivo and indicates adipogenesis in progress in vivo. J Mol Endocrinol. 2003;30(3):369–80.
53. Kumar S, Nadeem S, Stan MN, Coenen M, Bahn RS. A stimulatory TSH receptor antibody enhances adipogenesis via phosphoinositide 3-kinase activation in orbital preadipocytes from patients with Graves' ophthalmopathy. J Mol Endocrinol. 2011;46(3):155–63.
54. Tsui S, Naik V, Hoa N, Hwang CJ, Afifiyan NF, Sinha Hikim A, et al. Evidence for an association between thyroid-stimulating hormone and insulin-like growth factor 1 receptors: a tale of two antigens implicated in Graves' disease. J Immunol. 2008;181(6):4397–405.
55. Kohn LD, Alvarez F, Marcocci C, Kohn AD, Corda D, Hoffman WE, et al. Monoclonal antibody studies defining the origin and properties of autoantibodies in Graves' disease. Ann N Y Acad Sci. 1986;475:157–73.
56. Kumar S, Iyer S, Bauer H, Coenen M, Bahn RS. A stimulatory thyrotropin receptor antibody enhances hyaluronic acid synthesis in graves' orbital fibroblasts: inhibition by an IGF-I receptor blocking antibody. J Clin Endocrinol Metab. 2012;97(5):1681–7.
57. McKeag D, Lane C, Lazarus JH, Baldeschi L, Boboridis K, Dickinson AJ, et al. Clinical features of dysthyroid optic neuropathy: a European Group on Graves' Orbitopathy (EUGOGO) survey. Br J Ophthalmol. 2007;91(4):455–8.
58. Trobe JD, Glaser JS, Laflamme P. Dysthyroid optic neuropathy. Clinical profile and rationale for management. Arch Ophthalmol. 1978;96(7):1199–209.
59. Miller NR, Walsh FB, Hoyt WF. Walsh and Hoyt's clinical neuro-ophthalmology. 6th ed. Philadelphia: Lippincott Williams & Wilkins; 2005.
60. Day RM, Carroll FD. Optic nerve involvement associated with thyroid dysfunction. Trans Am Ophthalmol Soc. 1961;59:220–38.
61. Henderson JW. Optic neuropathy of exophthalmic goiter (Graves' disease). AMA Arch Ophthalmol. 1958;59(4):471–80.
62. Hedges Jr TR, Scheie HG. Visual field defects in exophthalmos associated with thyroid disease. AMA Arch Ophthalmol. 1955;54(6):885–92.
63. Igersheimer J. Visual changes in progressive exophthalmos. AMA Arch Ophthalmol. 1955;53(1):94–104.
64. McKeage K. Treatment options for the management of diabetic painful neuropathy: best current evidence. Curr Opin Neurol. 2007;20(5):553–7.

65. Muller-Forell W, Kahaly GJ. Neuroimaging of Graves' orbitopathy. Best Pract Res Clin Endocrinol Metab. 2012;26(3):259–71.

66. Bartalena L, Baldeschi L, Dickinson A, Eckstein A, Kendall-Taylor P, Marcocci C, et al. Consensus statement of the European Group on Graves' orbitopathy (EUGOGO) on management of GO. Eur J Endocrinol. 2008;158(3):273–85.

67. Bartley GB, Fatourechi V, Kadrmas EF, Jacobsen SJ, Ilstrup DM, Garrity JA, et al. Long-term follow-up of Graves ophthalmopathy in an incidence cohort. Ophthalmology. 1996;103(6):958–62.

68. Perros P, Kendall-Taylor P. Natural history of thyroid eye disease. Thyroid. 1998;8(5):423–5.

69. Neigel JM, Rootman J, Belkin RI, Nugent RA, Drance SM, Beattie CW, et al. Dysthyroid optic neuropathy. The crowded orbital apex syndrome. Ophthalmology. 1988;95(11):1515–21.

70. Werner SC. Modification of the classification of the eye changes of Graves' disease: recommendations of the Ad Hoc Committee of the American Thyroid Association. J Clin Endocrinol Metab. 1977;44(1):203–4.

71. Rundle FF, Wilson CW. Development and course of exophthalmos and ophthalmoplegia in Graves' disease with special reference to the effect of thyroidectomy. Clin Sci. 1945;5(3–4):177–94.

72. Mourits MP, Prummel MF, Wiersinga WM, Koornneef L. Clinical activity score as a guide in the management of patients with Graves' ophthalmopathy. Clin Endocrinol (Oxf). 1997;47(1):9–14.

73. Dolman PJ, Rootman J. VISA Classification for Graves orbitopathy. Ophthal Plast Reconstr Surg. 2006;22(5):319–24.

74. Wiersinga WM. Management of Graves' ophthalmopathy. Nat Clin Pract Endocrinol Metab. 2007;3(5):396–404.

75. Bartalena L. Prevention of Graves' ophthalmopathy. Best Pract Res Clin Endocrinol Metab. 2012;26(3):371–9.

76. Prummel MF, Wiersinga WM. Smoking and risk of Graves' disease. JAMA. 1993;269(4):479–82.

77. Bartalena L, Marcocci C, Tanda ML, Manetti L, Dell'Unto E, Bartolomei MP, et al. Cigarette smoking and treatment outcomes in Graves ophthalmopathy. Ann Intern Med. 1998;129(8):632–5.

78. Eckstein A, Quadbeck B, Mueller G, Rettenmeier AW, Hoermann R, Mann K, et al. Impact of smoking on the response to treatment of thyroid associated ophthalmopathy. Br J Ophthalmol. 2003;87(6):773–6.

79. Kalmann R, Mourits MP. Diabetes mellitus: a risk factor in patients with Graves' orbitopathy. Br J Ophthalmol. 1999;83(4):463–5.

80. Prummel MF, Wiersinga WM, Mourits MP, Koornneef L, Berghout A, van der Gaag R. Effect of abnormal thyroid function on the severity of Graves' ophthalmopathy. Arch Intern Med. 1990;150(5):1098–101.

81. Tallstedt L, Lundell G, Torring O, Wallin G, Ljunggren JG, Blomgren H, et al. Occurrence of ophthalmopathy after treatment for Graves' hyperthyroidism. The Thyroid Study Group. N Engl J Med. 1992;326(26):1733–8.

82. Bartalena L, Marcocci C, Bogazzi F, Manetti L, Tanda ML, Dell'Unto E, et al. Relation between therapy for hyperthyroidism and the course of Graves' ophthalmopathy. N Engl J Med. 1998;338(2):73–8.

83. Traisk F, Tallstedt L, Abraham-Nordling M, Andersson T, Berg G, Calissendorff J, et al. Thyroid-associated ophthalmopathy after treatment for Graves' hyperthyroidism with antithyroid drugs or iodine-131. J Clin Endocrinol Metab. 2009;94(10):3700–7.

84. Wiersinga WM. Autoimmunity in Graves' ophthalmopathy: the result of an unfortunate marriage between TSH receptors and IGF-1 receptors? J Clin Endocrinol Metab. 2011;96(8):2386–94.

85. Bartalena L. The dilemma of how to manage Graves' hyperthyroidism in patients with associated orbitopathy. J Clin Endocrinol Metab. 2011;96(3):592–9.

86. Menconi F, Profilo MA, Leo M, Sisti E, Altea MA, Rocchi R, et al. Spontaneous improvement of untreated mild graves' ophthalmopathy: Rundle's curve revisited. Thyroid. 2014;24(1):60–6.

87. Wiersinga WM. Quality of life in Graves' ophthalmopathy. Best Pract Res Clin Endocrinol Metab. 2012;26(3):359–70.

88. Marcocci C, Marino M. Treatment of mild, moderate-to-severe and very severe Graves' orbitopathy. Best Pract Res Clin Endocrinol Metab. 2012;26(3):325–37.

89. Marcocci C, Kahaly GJ, Krassas GE, Bartalena L, Prummel M, Stahl M, et al. Selenium and the course of mild Graves' orbitopathy. N Engl J Med. 2011;364(20):1920–31.

90. Bartalena L, Pinchera A, Marcocci C. Management of Graves' ophthalmopathy: reality and perspectives. Endocr Rev. 2000;21(2):168–99.

91. Zang S, Ponto KA, Kahaly GJ. Clinical review: intravenous glucocorticoids for Graves' orbitopathy: efficacy and morbidity. J Clin Endocrinol Metab. 2011;96(2):320–32.

92. Smith TJ. Dexamethasone regulation of glycosaminoglycan synthesis in cultured human skin fibroblasts. Similar effects of glucocorticoid and thyroid hormones. J Clin Invest. 1984;74(6):2157–63.

93. Marcocci C, Bartalena L, Tanda ML, Manetti L, Dell'Unto E, Rocchi R, et al. Comparison of the effectiveness and tolerability of intravenous or oral glucocorticoids associated with orbital radiotherapy in the management of severe Graves' ophthalmopathy: results of a prospective, single-blind, randomized study. J Clin Endocrinol Metab. 2001;86(8):3562–7.

94. Kahaly GJ, Pitz S, Hommel G, Dittmar M. Randomized, single blind trial of intravenous versus oral steroid monotherapy in Graves' orbitopathy. J Clin Endocrinol Metab. 2005;90(9):5234–40.

95. Curro N, Covelli D, Vannucchi G, Campi I, Pirola G, Simonetta S, et al. Therapeutic Outcomes of

High-Dose Intravenous Steroids in the Treatment of Dysthyroid Optic Neuropathy. Thyroid. 2014;24:897–905.

96. Wakelkamp IM, Baldeschi L, Saeed P, Mourits MP, Prummel MF, Wiersinga WM. Surgical or medical decompression as a first-line treatment of optic neuropathy in Graves' ophthalmopathy? A randomized controlled trial. Clin Endocrinol (Oxf). 2005;63(3):323–8.

97. Bartalena L, Marcocci C, Chiovato L, Laddaga M, Lepri G, Andreani D, et al. Orbital cobalt irradiation combined with systemic corticosteroids for Graves' ophthalmopathy: comparison with systemic corticosteroids alone. J Clin Endocrinol Metab. 1983;56(6):1139–44.

98. Marcocci C, Bartalena L, Bogazzi F, Bruno-Bossio G, Lepri A, Pinchera A. Orbital radiotherapy combined with high dose systemic glucocorticoids for Graves' ophthalmopathy is more effective than radiotherapy alone: results of a prospective randomized study. J Endocrinol Invest. 1991;14(10):853–60.

99. Weissel M, Hauff W. Fatal liver failure after high-dose glucocorticoid pulse therapy in a patient with severe thyroid eye disease. Thyroid. 2000;10(6):521.

100. Marino M, Morabito E, Brunetto MR, Bartalena L, Pinchera A, Marocci C. Acute and severe liver damage associated with intravenous glucocorticoid pulse therapy in patients with Graves' ophthalmopathy. Thyroid. 2004;14(5):403–6.

101. Lendorf ME, Rasmussen AK, Fledelius HC, Feldt-Rasmussen U. Cardiovascular and cerebrovascular events in temporal relationship to intravenous glucocorticoid pulse therapy in patients with severe endocrine ophthalmopathy. Thyroid. 2009;19(12):1431–2.

102. Gursoy A, Cesur M, Erdogan MF, Corapcioglu D, Kamel N. New-onset acute heart failure after intravenous glucocorticoid pulse therapy in a patient with Graves' ophthalmopathy. Endocrine. 2006;29(3):513–6.

103. Salvi M, Vannucchi G, Sbrozzi F, Del Castello AB, Carnevali A, Fargion S, et al. Onset of autoimmune hepatitis during intravenous steroid therapy for thyroid-associated ophthalmopathy in a patient with Hashimoto's thyroiditis: case report. Thyroid. 2004;14(8):631–4.

104. Tigas S, Papachilleos P, Ligkros N, Andrikoula M, Tsatsoulis A. Hypokalemic paralysis following administration of intravenous methylprednisolone in a patient with Graves' thyrotoxicosis and ophthalmopathy. Hormones (Athens). 2011;10(4):313–6.

105. Wichary H, Gasinska T. Methylprednisolone and hepatotoxicity in Graves' ophthalmopathy. Thyroid. 2012;22(1):64–9.

106. Bartalena L, Marcocci C, Tanda ML, Rocchi R, Mazzi B, Barbesino G, et al. Orbital radiotherapy for Graves' ophthalmopathy. Thyroid. 2002;12(3):245–50.

107. Dolman PJ, Rath S. Orbital radiotherapy for thyroid eye disease. Curr Opin Ophthalmol. 2012;23(5):427–32.

108. Tanda ML, Bartalena L. Efficacy and safety of orbital radiotherapy for graves' orbitopathy. J Clin Endocrinol Metab. 2012;97(11):3857–65.

109. Ohtsuka K, Sato A, Kawaguchi S, Hashimoto M, Suzuki Y. Effect of steroid pulse therapy with and without orbital radiotherapy on Graves' ophthalmopathy. Am J Ophthalmol. 2003;135(3):285–90.

110. Prummel MF, Mourits MP, Blank L, Berghout A, Koornneef L, Wiersinga WM. Randomized double-blind trial of prednisone versus radiotherapy in Graves' ophthalmopathy. Lancet. 1993;342(8877):949–54.

111. Marcocci C, Bartalena L, Rocchi R, Marino M, Menconi F, Morabito E, et al. Long-term safety of orbital radiotherapy for Graves' ophthalmopathy. J Clin Endocrinol Metab. 2003;88(8):3561–6.

112. Wakelkamp IM, Tan H, Saeed P, Schlingemann RO, Verbraak FD, Blank LE, et al. Orbital irradiation for Graves' ophthalmopathy: is it safe? A long-term follow-up study. Ophthalmology. 2004;111(8):1557–62.

113. Trokel S, Kazim M, Moore S. Orbital fat removal. Decompression for Graves orbitopathy. Ophthalmology. 1993;100(5):674–82.

114. Kahaly GJ, Rosler HP, Pitz S, Hommel G. Low-versus high-dose radiotherapy for Graves' ophthalmopathy: a randomized, single blind trial. J Clin Endocrinol Metab. 2000;85(1):102–8.

115. Gerling J, Kommerell G, Henne K, Laubenberger J, Schulte-Monting J, Fells P. Retrobulbar irradiation for thyroid-associated orbitopathy: double-blind comparison between 2.4 and 16 Gy. Int J Radiat Oncol Biol Phys. 2003;55(1):182–9.

116. Snijders-Keilholz A, De Keizer RJ, Goslings BM, Van Dam EW, Jansen JT, Broerse JJ. Probable risk of tumour induction after retro-orbital irradiation for Graves' ophthalmopathy. Radiother Oncol. 1996;38(1):69–71.

117. Paridaens D, van den Bosch WA, van der Loos TL, Krenning EP, van Hagen PM. The effect of etanercept on Graves' ophthalmopathy: a pilot study. Eye (Lond). 2005;19(12):1286–9.

118. Prummel MF, Mourits MP, Berghout A, Krenning EP, van der Gaag R, Koornneef L, et al. Prednisone and cyclosporine in the treatment of severe Graves' ophthalmopathy. N Engl J Med. 1989;321(20):1353–9.

119. Rajendram R, Lee RW, Potts MJ, Rose GE, Jain R, Olver JM, et al. Protocol for the combined immunosuppression & radiotherapy in thyroid eye disease (CIRTED) trial: a multi-centre, double-masked, factorial randomised controlled trial. Trials. 2008;9:6.

120. Bartalena L, Lai A, Compri E, Marcocci C, Tanda ML. Novel immunomodulating agents for Graves orbitopathy. Ophthal Plast Reconstr Surg. 2008;24(4):251–6.

121. Chang S, Perry JD, Kosmorsky GS, Braun WE. Rapamycin for treatment of refractory dysthyroid compressive optic neuropathy. Ophthal Plast Reconstr Surg. 2007;23(3):225–6.

122. Kahaly G, Schrezenmeir J, Krause U, Schweikert B, Meuer S, Muller W, et al. Ciclosporin and predni-

sone v. prednisone in treatment of Graves' ophthalmopathy: a controlled, randomized and prospective study. Eur J Clin Invest. 1986;16(5):415–22.

123. Salvi M, Vannucchi G, Beck-Peccoz P. Potential utility of rituximab for Graves' orbitopathy. J Clin Endocrinol Metab. 2013;98(11):4291–9.

124. Salvi M, Vannucchi G, Campi I, Curro N, Dazzi D, Simonetta S, et al. Treatment of Graves' disease and associated ophthalmopathy with the anti-CD20 monoclonal antibody rituximab: an open study. Eur J Endocrinol. 2007;156(1):33–40.

125. Salvi M, Vannucchi G, Curro N, Introna M, Rossi S, Bonara P, et al. Small dose of rituximab for graves orbitopathy: new insights into the mechanism of action. Arch Ophthalmol. 2012;130(1):122–4.

126. Salvi M, Vannucchi G, Campi I, Curro N, Simonetta S, Covelli D, et al. Rituximab treatment in a patient with severe thyroid-associated ophthalmopathy: effects on orbital lymphocytic infiltrates. Clin Immunol. 2009;131(2):360–5.

127. Salvi M, Vannucchi G, Campi I, Rossi S, Bonara P, Sbrozzi F, et al. Efficacy of rituximab treatment for thyroid-associated ophthalmopathy as a result of intraorbital B-cell depletion in one patient unresponsive to steroid immunosuppression. Eur J Endocrinol. 2006;154(4):511–7.

128. El Fassi D, Nielsen CH, Hasselbalch HC, Hegedus L. Treatment-resistant severe, active Graves' ophthalmopathy successfully treated with B lymphocyte depletion. Thyroid. 2006;16(7):709–10.

129. Khanna D, Chong KK, Afifiyan NF, Hwang CJ, Lee DK, Garneau HC, et al. Rituximab treatment of patients with severe, corticosteroid-resistant thyroid-associated ophthalmopathy. Ophthalmology. 2010;117(1):133–9 e2.

130. Krassas GE, Stafilidou A, Boboridis KG. Failure of rituximab treatment in a case of severe thyroid ophthalmopathy unresponsive to steroids. Clin Endocrinol (Oxf). 2010;72(6):853–5.

131. Silkiss RZ, Reier A, Coleman M, Lauer SA. Rituximab for thyroid eye disease. Ophthal Plast Reconstr Surg. 2010;26(5):310–4.

132. Madaschi S, Rossini A, Formenti I, Lampasona V, Marzoli SB, Cammarata G, et al. Treatment of thyroid-associated orbitopathy with rituximab–a novel therapy for an old disease: case report and literature review. Endocr Pract. 2010;16(4):677–85.

133. Eckstein A, Schittkowski M, Esser J. Surgical treatment of Graves' ophthalmopathy. Best Pract Res Clin Endocrinol Metab. 2012;26(3):339–58.

134. Otto AJ, Koornneef L, Mourits MP, Deen-van Leeuwen L. Retrobulbar pressures measured during surgical decompression of the orbit. Br J Ophthalmol. 1996;80(12):1042–5.

135. Goldberg RA. The evolving paradigm of orbital decompression surgery. Arch Ophthalmol. 1998;116(1):95–6.

136. Liao SL, Chang TC, Lin LL. Transcaruncular orbital decompression: an alternate procedure for Graves ophthalmopathy with compressive optic neuropathy. Am J Ophthalmol. 2006;141(5):810–8.

137. McCann JD, Goldberg RA, Anderson RL, Burroughs JR, Ben Simon GJ. Medial wall decompression for optic neuropathy but lateral wall decompression with fat removal for non vision-threatening indications. Am J Ophthalmol. 2006;141(5):916–7.

138. Metson R, Pletcher SD. Endoscopic orbital and optic nerve decompression. Otolaryngol Clin North Am. 2006;39(3):551–61, ix.

139. Siracuse-Lee DE, Kazim M. Orbital decompression: current concepts. Curr Opin Ophthalmol. 2002;13(5):310–6.

140. Graham SM, Brown CL, Carter KD, Song A, Nerad JA. Medial and lateral orbital wall surgery for balanced decompression in thyroid eye disease. Laryngoscope. 2003;113(7):1206–9.

141. Olivari N. Transpalpebral decompression of endocrine ophthalmopathy (Graves' disease) by removal of intraorbital fat: experience with 147 operations over 5 years. Plast Reconstr Surg. 1991;87(4):627–41; discussion 42–3.

142. Boboridis KG, Bunce C. Surgical orbital decompression for thyroid eye disease. Cochrane Database Syst Rev. 2011;12, CD007630.

143. O'Malley MR, Meyer DR. Transconjunctival fat removal combined with conservative medial wall/floor orbital decompression for Graves orbitopathy. Ophthal Plast Reconstr Surg. 2009;25(3):206–10.

144. Unal M, Leri F, Konuk O, Hasanreisoglu B. Balanced orbital decompression combined with fat removal in Graves ophthalmopathy: do we really need to remove the third wall? Ophthal Plast Reconstr Surg. 2003;19(2):112–8.

145. Kazim M, Trokel SL, Acaroglu G, Elliott A. Reversal of dysthyroid optic neuropathy following orbital fat decompression. Br J Ophthalmol. 2000;84(6):600–5.

146. Goldberg RA, Perry JD, Hortaleza V, Tong JT. Strabismus after balanced medial plus lateral wall versus lateral wall only orbital decompression for dysthyroid orbitopathy. Ophthal Plast Reconstr Surg. 2000;16(4):271–7.

147. Garrity JA, Fatourechi V, Bergstralh EJ, Bartley GB, Beatty CW, DeSanto LW, et al. Results of transantral orbital decompression in 428 patients with severe Graves' ophthalmopathy. Am J Ophthalmol. 1993;116(5):533–47.

148. Ben Simon GJ, Wang L, McCann JD, Goldberg RA. Primary-gaze diplopia in patients with thyroid-related orbitopathy undergoing deep lateral orbital decompression with intraconal fat debulking: a retrospective analysis of treatment outcome. Thyroid. 2004;14(5):379–83.

149. Dollinger J. Die Druckentlastung der Augenhöhle durch Entfernung der äusseren Orbitawand bei hochgradigenvExophthalmos und konsekutiver Hornhauterkrankungen. Dtsch Med Wochenschr. 1911;37:1988–90.

150. Kroll AJ, Casten VG. Dysthyroid exophthalmos. Palliation by lateral orbital decompression. Arch Ophthalmol. 1966;76(2):205–10.

151. Goldberg RA, Weinberg DA, Shorr N, Wirta D. Maximal, three-wall, orbital decompression through

a coronal approach. Ophthalmic Surg Lasers. 1997;28(10):832–43.

152. McCord Jr CD. Current trends in orbital decompression. Ophthalmology. 1985;92(1):21–33.

153. Shorr N, Baylis HI, Goldberg RA, Perry JD. Transcaruncular approach to the medial orbit and orbital apex. Ophthalmology. 2000;107(8):1459–63.

154. Chang EL, Bernardino CR, Rubin PA. Transcaruncular orbital decompression for management of compressive optic neuropathy in thyroid-related orbitopathy. Plast Reconstr Surg. 2003;112(3):739–47.

155. Baldeschi L. Correction of lid retraction and exophthalmos. Dev Ophthalmol. 2008;41:103–26.

156. Cansiz H, Yilmaz S, Karaman E, Ogreden S, Acioglu E, Sekercioglu N, et al. Three-wall orbital decompression superiority to 2-wall orbital decompression in thyroid-associated ophthalmopathy. J Oral Maxillofac Surg. 2006;64(5):763–9.

157. Douglas RS, Goldberg RA, Smith TJ. A symposium on thyroid-associated ophthalmopathy, also known as Graves' orbitopathy at the Jules Stein Eye Institute at the University of California, Los Angeles. Thyroid. 2008;18(9):931.

158. Paridaens DA, Verhoeff K, Bouwens D, van Den Bosch WA. Transconjunctival orbital decompression in Graves' ophthalmopathy: lateral wall approach ab interno. Br J Ophthalmol. 2000;84(7):775–81.

159. Boulos PR, Hardy I. Thyroid-associated orbitopathy: a clinicopathologic and therapeutic review. Curr Opin Ophthalmol. 2004;15(5):389–400.

160. Trokel SL, Cooper WC. Symposium: extraocular muscle problems associated with graves' disease. Orbital decompression: effect on motility and globe position. Ophthalmology. 1979;86(12):2064–70.

161. Abramoff MD, Kalmann R, de Graaf ME, Stilma JS, Mourits MP. Rectus extraocular muscle paths and decompression surgery for Graves orbitopathy: mechanism of motility disturbances. Invest Ophthalmol Vis Sci. 2002;43(2):300–7.

162. Inoue Y, Tsuboi T, Kouzaki A, Maeda T, Inoue T. Ophthalmic surgery in dysthyroid ophthalmopathy. Thyroid. 2002;12(3):257–63.

163. Seiff SR, Tovilla JL, Carter SR, Choo PH. Modified orbital decompression for dysthyroid orbitopathy. Ophthal Plast Reconstr Surg. 2000;16(1):62–6.

164. Millar MJ, Maloof AJ. The application of stereotactic navigation surgery to orbital decompression for thyroid-associated orbitopathy. Eye (Lond). 2009;23(7):1565–71.

165. Kikkawa DO, Cruz Jr RC, Christian WK, Rikkers S, Weinreb RN, Levi L, et al. Botulinum A toxin injection for restrictive myopathy of thyroid-related

orbitopathy: effects on intraocular pressure. Am J Ophthalmol. 2003;135(4):427–31.

166. Uddin JM, Davies PD. Treatment of upper eyelid retraction associated with thyroid eye disease with subconjunctival botulinum toxin injection. Ophthalmology. 2002;109(6):1183–7.

167. Wabbels B, Forl M. Botulinum toxin treatment for crocodile tears, spastic entropion and for dysthyroid upper eyelid retraction. Ophthalmologe. 2007;104(9):771–6.

168. Shih MJ, Liao SL, Kuo KT, Smith TJ, Chuang LM. Molecular pathology of Muller's muscle in Graves' ophthalmopathy. J Clin Endocrinol Metab. 2006;91(3):1159–67.

169. Chang HS, Lee D, Taban M, Douglas RS, Goldberg RA. "En-glove" lysis of lower eyelid retractors with AlloDerm and dermis-fat grafts in lower eyelid retraction surgery. Ophthal Plast Reconstr Surg. 2011;27(2):137–41.

170. Cohen MS, Shorr N. Eyelid reconstruction with hard palate mucosa grafts. Ophthal Plast Reconstr Surg. 1992;8(3):183–95.

171. Doxanas MT, Dryden RM. The use of sclera in the treatment of dysthyroid eyelid retraction. Ophthalmology. 1981;88(9):887–94.

172. Feldman KA, Putterman AM, Farber MD. Surgical treatment of thyroid-related lower eyelid retraction: a modified approach. Ophthal Plast Reconstr Surg. 1992;8(4):278–86.

173. McCord C, Nahai FR, Codner MA, Nahai F, Hester TR. Use of porcine acellular dermal matrix (Enduragen) grafts in eyelids: a review of 69 patients and 129 eyelids. Plast Reconstr Surg. 2008;122(4):1206–13.

174. Mourits MP, Koornneef L. Lid lengthening by sclera interposition for eyelid retraction in Graves' ophthalmopathy. Br J Ophthalmol. 1991;75(6):344–7.

175. Oestreicher JH, Pang NK, Liao W. Treatment of lower eyelid retraction by retractor release and posterior lamellar grafting: an analysis of 659 eyelids in 400 patients. Ophthal Plast Reconstr Surg. 2008;24(3):207–12.

176. Olver JM, Rose GE, Khaw PT, Collin JR. Correction of lower eyelid retraction in thyroid eye disease: a randomised controlled trial of retractor tenotomy with adjuvant antimetabolite versus scleral graft. Br J Ophthalmol. 1998;82(2):174–80.

177. Tan J, Olver J, Wright M, Maini R, Neoh C, Dickinson AJ. The use of porous polyethylene (Medpor) lower eyelid spacers in lid heightening and stabilisation. Br J Ophthalmol. 2004;88(9):1197–200.

178. Waller RR. Lower eyelid retraction: management. Ophthalmic Surg. 1978;9(3):41–7.

Printing and Binding: Stürtz GmbH, Würzburg